WITHDRAWN

FROM
UNIVERSITIES
AT
MEDWAY
LIBRARY

D1339319

NWCHW
08008103

For Elsevier:

Commissioning Editor: Robert Edwards
Development Editor: Rebecca Gleave
Project Manager: Jess Thompson
Design Direction: George Ajayi
Illustrator: Precision Illustration
Illustration Manager: Merlyn Harvey

eye essentials

8011195

diabetes and the eye

Chris Steele BSc (Hons) FCOptom DCLP DipOC FBCLA
Consultant Optometrist, Head of Optometry, Sunderland Eye Infirmary, Sunderland, UK

David Steel MBBS FRCOpth
Consultant Opthalmologist, Sunderland Eye Infirmary, Sunderland, UK

Colin Waine OBE MBBS FRCGP FRCPath
School of Health, Natural and Social Sciences, Priestman Building, Sunderland University, Sunderland, UK

SERIES EDITORS

Sandip Doshi PhD MCOptom
Optometrist in private practice, Hove, East Sussex, UK
Examiner, College of Optometrists, London, UK
Formerly Clinical Editor, Optician

William Harvey MCOptom
Visiting Clinician and Director of Visual Impairment Clinic, City University, London, UK
Professional Programme Tutor for Boots Opticians Ltd
Clinical Editor, Optician, Reed Business Information, Sutton, UK

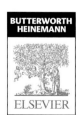

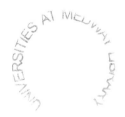

BUTTERWORTH
HEINEMANN

ELSEVIER   EDINBURGH LONDON NEW YORK OXFORD
PHILADELPHIA ST LOUIS SYDNEY TORONTO 2008

BUTTERWORTH
HEINEMANN
ELSEVIER

© 2008, Elsevier Limited. All rights reserved.

No part of this publication may be reproduced, stored in a retrieval system, or transmitted in any form or by any means, electronic, mechanical, photocopying, recording or otherwise, without the prior permission of the Publishers. Permissions may be sought directly from Elsevier's Health Sciences Rights Department, 1600 John F. Kennedy Boulevard, Suite 1800, Philadelphia, PA 19103-2899, USA: phone:(+1) 215 239 3804: fax: (+1) 215 239 3805; or, e-mail: healthpermissions@elsevier.com. You may also complete your request on-line via the Elsevier homepage (http://www.elsevier.com), by selecting 'Support and contact' and then 'Copyright and Permission'.

First published 2008
  Reprinted 2008

ISBN 978-0-08-045307-1

British Library Cataloguing in Publication Data
A catalogue record for this book is available from the British Library

Library of Congress Cataloging in Publication Data
A catalog record for this book is available from the Library of Congress

Note
Knowledge and best practice in this field are constantly changing. As new research and experience broaden our knowledge, changes in practice, treatment and drug therapy may become necessary or appropriate. Readers are advised to check the most current information provided (i) on procedures featured or (ii) by the manufacturer of each product to be administered, to verify the recommended dose or formula, the method and duration of administration, and contraindications. It is the responsibility of the practitioner, relying on their own experience and knowledge of the patient, to make diagnoses, to determine dosages and the best treatment for each individual patient, and to take all appropriate safety precautions.
To the fullest extent of the law, neither the publisher nor the editors assumes any liability for any injury and/or damage.

The Publisher

Working together to grow
libraries in developing countries

www.elsevier.com | www.bookaid.org | www.sabre.org

ELSEVIER   BOOK AID
            International   Sabre Foundation

ELSEVIER   your source for books,
            journals and multimedia
            in the health sciences
www.elsevierhealth.com

The
publisher's
policy is to use
paper manufactured
from sustainable forests

Printed in China

Contents

UNIVERSITIES AT MEDWAY
2 2 MAY 2009
DRILL HALL LIBRARY

Foreword

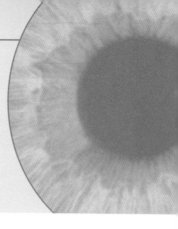

Eye Essentials is a series of books intended to cover the core skills required by the eye care practitioner in general and/or specialized practice. It consists of books covering a wide range of topics, ranging from: routine eye examination to assessment and management of low vision; assessment and investigative techniques to digital imaging; case reports and law to contact lenses.

Authors known for their interest and expertise in their particular subject have contributed books to this series. The reader will know many of them, as they have published widely within their respective fields. Each author has addressed key topics in their subject in a practical rather than theoretical approach, hence each book has a particular relevance to everyday practice.

Each book in the series follows a similar format and has been designed to enable the reader to ascertain information easily and quickly. Each chapter has been produced in a user-friendly format, thus providing the reader with a rapid-reference book that is easy to use in the consulting room or in the practitioner's free time.

Optometry and dispensing optics are continually developing professions, with the emphasis in each being redefined as we learn more from research and as technology stamps its mark. The *Eye Essentials* series is particularly relevant to the practitioner's requirements and as such will appeal to students, graduates sitting professional examinations and qualified practitioners alike. We hope you enjoy reading these books as much as we have enjoyed producing them.

Sandip Doshi
Bill Harvey

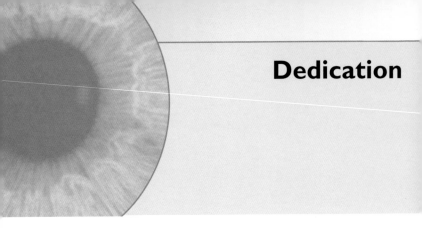

Dedication

This book is dedicated to Sam, Isabel, Madeleine and Imogen Steele, Rachel and Ben Steel and Jennifer and Anna Waine – our collective young children.

Acknowledgements

We would like to thank Helen Bone, Identifying Retinopathy in Sunderland (IRIS) Team Leader for all her help preparing the manuscripts. Thank you to the IRIS Retinal Screening Team (Nicola Coyles, Russell Martin, Vikki Bradley and Jan Lorraine) as well as Terri Ainley, Medical Photographer, Sunderland Eye Infirmary for all their help with collating images for this book. Thank you to Mr Jim Deady, Consultant Ophthalmologist, Sunderland Eye Infirmary for his guidance and clinical input.

We are grateful to The Institute of Optometry for agreeing to allow us to include material previously written by ourselves for the diabetes module of the Ocular Therapeutics Supplementary and Additional Supply Course. Finally my special thanks to Afroditi Sideropoulou for all her help and support during the writing of this book.

Chris Steele

Introduction

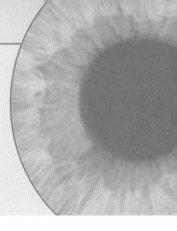

Diabetes is recognized as a group of heterogeneous disorders with the common elements of hyperglycaemia and glucose intolerance due to insulin deficiency, impaired effectiveness of insulin action, or both. The underlying causes for this hyperglycaemia are either an absolute or relative lack of the hormone insulin. This is caused by the pancreas not producing insulin or insufficient insulin action to meet the body's requirements.

We are currently witnessing a worldwide epidemic of diabetes with the current prevalence being approximately 200 million people affected around the world. Diabetes mellitus and lesser forms of glucose intolerance, particularly impaired glucose tolerance (IGT), can now be found in almost every population in the world and epidemiological evidence suggests that, without effective prevention and control programmes, diabetes will likely continue to increase globally. In fact the prevalence of diabetes is expected to double by 2025.

The two main types of diabetes are type 1 (formerly called 'insulin dependent') and type 2 (formerly called 'non-insulin dependent') diabetes. Type 1 diabetes is the most common chronic childhood disease in developed nations and the clinical presentation can vary with age. The predominant cause of hyperglycaemia in type 1 diabetes is the autoimmune destruction of the pancreatic beta cells, which leads to absolute dependence on insulin treatment and a high rate of complications typically occurring at relatively young ages.

Type 2 diabetes is characterized by insulin resistance and relative insulin deficiency, either of which may be present at the time that diabetes becomes clinically manifest. The specific reasons for the development of these abnormalities are still not yet fully understood but are certainly multi-factorial. Type 2 diabetes is often, but not always, associated with obesity, which itself can cause insulin resistance and lead to hyperglycaemia. It is strongly familial, but major susceptibility genes have as yet not been identified.

Type 2 diabetes is the most common type, accounting for approximately 85% of cases in most Caucasian populations and western countries and up to 95% of diabetes in developing countries. The main reason for this is thought to be because of these developing countries adopting a western life style.

In virtually every developed society, diabetes is one of the leading causes of blindness, renal failure and lower limb amputation. It is also now one of the leading causes of death through its effects on cardiovascular disease (70–80% of people with diabetes die of cardiovascular disease). The main relevance of diabetes complications from a public health perspective is the relationship with human suffering and disability, and the huge socio-economic costs through premature morbidity and mortality.

In the first five chapters, the different types of diabetes are discussed and how these conditions are diagnosed and currently treated. The systemic manifestations of the diabetes are also explained and how these various conditions can be managed by both medics and other healthcare professionals. The aim has been to provide a comprehensive clinical guide with a practical approach to the management of diabetes to what is actually a very complex condition. This book is intended as an essential introductory reference source for optometrists, medical students, junior doctors and other healthcare professionals, that is written in such a way as to give the busy clinician the practical information they need without overwhelming them with too much complex detail. For those readers wishing to explore particular areas of interest, there are comprehensive further reading lists at the end of each chapter.

In the latter five chapters, the effects of diabetes on the eye are reviewed along with treatment strategies, with Chapter 6 dedicated to the pathophysiology of diabetic retinopathy. In Chapter 7 the clinical features of non-proliferative (background) diabetic retinopathy and pre-proliferative and proliferative retinopathy are discussed as well as the different forms of diabetic maculopathy. The treatments available for diabetic retinopathy have been expanding in recent years. Although retinal photocoagulation and vitrectomy are effective treatments for diabetic retinopathy they do not address the fundamental disease processes associated with the occurrence of retinopathy. There are now a number of new treatments being developed for diabetic retinopathy and this is a particularly exciting area at present. These new medical treatments, laser technologies and surgical approaches are discussed in Chapter 8.

Diabetic retinopathy often presents alongside a wide range of other eye diseases which are discussed in Chapter 9. Cataracts are very common in diabetics and particular emphasis has been placed on discussing the importance of managing diabetic patients with cataracts in the most appropriate way according to the current evidence base.

It is now becoming increasingly evident that control of other systemic factors and the use of different systemic therapeutic agents are very important in controlling diabetic retinopathy progression. To effectively manage diabetic retinopathy, once it has been detected by means of an effective screening system, involves optimizing glucose control and managing the common systemic conditions associated with diabetes, e.g. hypertension, dyslipidaemia, anaemia and obstructive sleep apnoea. Managing the effects of diabetes on other organs is also vital — in particular renal impairment. Diabetic nephropathy is strongly associated with sight-threatening diabetic retinopathy. The control of systemic factors is discussed in Chapter 10.

In order to achieve a holistic level of care for diabetic patients requires multidisciplinary teamwork between optometrists, general practitioners, ophthalmologists, specialist diabetes nurses, hospital-based physicians and paramedical staff including podiatrists, dieticians and retinal screeners. Only by working

together, communicating effectively and also keeping the patient fully informed, will all the healthcare needs of the diabetic patient be tackled coherently and effectively. This book pulls together all the essential information on which to base sound clinical decisions when dealing with the needs of the diabetic patient.

Chris Steele

1
Epidemiology, classification and diagnostic criteria of diabetes mellitus

Type 1 and type 2 diabetes are worldwide disorders. They can occur at virtually any time of life and have a massive adverse impact on the health of individuals and on health economies (Fig. 1.1).

United Kingdom prevalence of diabetes

It is estimated that about 1.4 million people in the United Kingdom have diabetes. Of these:

- about 1.25 million have type 2 diabetes;
- 0.15 million have type 1 diabetes;
- it is estimated that there may be as many as one million people with undiagnosed type 2 diabetes — such is its insidious onset;
- a new patient is diagnosed with type 2 diabetes every 5 minutes.

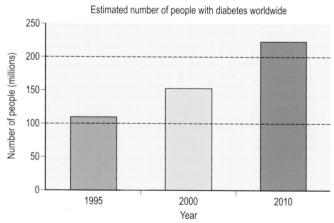

Fig. 1.1 Diabetes: an increasing global burden.

Type 2 diabetes

This is by far the commonest form of diabetes in the UK and indeed worldwide.

The risk factors for developing type 2 diabetes are:

- family history;
- obesity defined as BMI $>/= 30$ kg/m^2;
- increasing age;
- physical inactivity;
- high fat, energy dense diet;
- ethnicity — especially in the UK in people of Asian and Afro-Caribbean descent.

Type 1 diabetes

Genetic susceptibility may well play a part in the difference of prevalence in different parts of the world. It is highest in Scandinavia and lowest in Japan. Its prevalence rises with distance from the equator. Even in the British Isles, there is a marked variation. This varies from 6.8 per 100 000 in the Republic of Ireland to 19.8 per 100 000 in Scotland.

The incidence of type 1 diabetes has been increasing quite rapidly over the past 20 years for reasons which have not yet been adequately explained (Fig. 1.2). However, it does appear that ethnic groups emigrating to westernized societies assume the prevalence of type 1 diabetes of the indigenous population (Figs. 1.3 and 1.4). This suggests an environmental influence. The peak incidence of type 1 diabetes is in the early teenage years for both girls and boys with a small male excess.

There is a seasonal variation in the incidence of type 1 diabetes; it is more common in the autumn and winter.

4

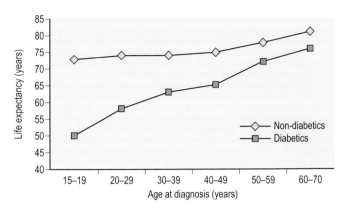

'Adults with diabetes have an annual mortality of about 5.4%, double the rate for non-diabetic adults. Life expectancy is decreased by 5–10 years'

Fig. 1.2 Life expectancy and diabetes.

The economic costs of diabetes (year 2000)

NHS diabetes expenditure £4 878 000 000 (9% of NHS budget) equivalent to:

Per week	£93 807 692
Per day	£13 401 098
Per hour	£558 379
Per minute	£9 306
Per second	£155

The major costs associated with diabetes relate to expenditure on the micro and macro-vascular complications affecting the eye, the kidney, the nervous system and the cardiovascular system.

Classification and diagnostic criteria

Diabetes mellitus is really a complex metabolic disorder in which there is persistent hyperglycaemia. Its manifestations impact on virtually every system in the body.

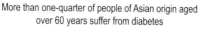

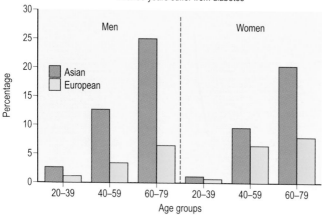

Fig. 1.3 Prevalence of diabetes in the UK Asian population.

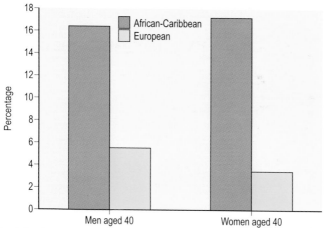

Fig. 1.4 Prevalence of diabetes in the UK African-Caribbean population.

Classification

Diabetes can be classified into the following types:

- **Type 1 diabetes**, formerly known as insulin-dependent diabetes mellitus (IDDM) or juvenile onset diabetes.

- **Type 2 diabetes**, formerly known as non-insulin dependent diabetes mellitus (NIDDM) or maturity onset diabetes (MOD).

Other types include:

- maturity onset diabetes in the young (MODY);
- genetic defects of insulin secretion which are quite rare;
- diseases of the exocrine pancreas, e.g. pancreatitis or carcinoma;
- drug- or chemical-induced diabetes — Alloxan;
- gestational diabetes mellitus (GDM).

Type 1 diabetes

In this condition there is an immune-mediated destruction of the pancreatic beta cells which produce insulin. It is characterized by an absolute deficiency of insulin and is normally of rapid onset with the characteristic symptoms of:

- thirst;
- polyuria;
- weight loss.

In the absence of effective treatment (exogenous insulin) it can rapidly progress to dehydration, diabetic keto-acidosis, coma and death. People with type 1 diabetes require insulin for their survival. They make up about 15% of the total diabetic population.

Type 2 diabetes

In this form of diabetes the main problems are insulin resistance and beta cell dysfunction. It is usually of insidious onset and people can have complications at diagnosis. Type 2 diabetes makes up about 85% of the total diabetic population so that it is by far the commonest form of diabetes. It is frequently associated with the overweight and obesity. In fact about 85% of people with type 2 diabetes are overweight or obese.

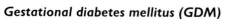

Gestational diabetes mellitus (GDM)

This is diabetes which develops during pregnancy, resolves after delivery but can recur in subsequent pregnancies.

Risk factors for developing GDM are obesity, previous history of still-birth or big babies and having previously had GDM. People who develop GDM are at increased risk of developing type 2 diabetes in later life. They are also at increased risk of developing hypertension. Asians and African-Caribbeans are particularly at risk.

Regarding the other forms of diabetes, genetic defects of insulin secretion are very rare. Of all diseases of the exocrine pancreas — the commonest is cystic fibrosis, others are carcinoma of the pancreas and pancreatitis.

Of the endocrinopathies, Cushing's disease and acromegally are examples.

Drug- or chemical-induced hypoglycaemia

Corticosteroids have by far the greatest impact on glucose tolerance of any groups of drugs. They act by increasing gluconeogenesis (the manufacture of glucose in the liver) and by increasing insulin resistance. The thiazide diuretics, commonly used in the treatment of hypertension and congestive heart failure, act by impairing insulin secretion.

Beta-blockers can impair glucose tolerance and thus exacerbate hyperglycaemia.

MODY clusters in families. There is a strong genetic component. The genetic components are complex and still being unravelled. Some forms seem to have an immunity to complications. In terms of everyday clinical practice, it is comparatively rare.

Diagnostic criteria

These are defined in Table 1.1. In asymptomatic patients two abnormal fasting values are required for diagnosis. There are two other important conditions:

- impaired fasting glucose (IFG);
- impaired glucose tolerance (IGT).

These are precursors of frank diabetes mellitus and people with them are at risk of developing type 2 diabetes. They are important not only because they are risk factors, but also because people with these conditions are at risk of developing the vascular complications associated with fully developed type 2 diabetes.

The World Health Organization criteria for these conditions are shown in Tables 1.2 and 1.3.

Table 1.1 WHO diagnostic criteria: diabetes mellitus

	Glucose concentration (mmol/l)		
	Whole blood venous	Whole blood capillary	Plasma venous
Diabetes mellitus			
Fasting[a]	≥6.1	≥6.1	≥7.0
or			
2-hour post-glucose load or both	≥10.0	≥11.1	≥11.1

[a]In asymptomatic patients two abnormal fasting values are required for diagnosis. World Health Organization. Report of a WHO consultation, 1999.

Table 1.2 WHO diagnostic criteria: impaired glucose tolerance (IGT)

	Glucose concentration (mmol/l)		
	Whole blood venous	Whole blood capillary	Plasma venous
Impaired glucose tolerance			
Fasting (if measured)	<6.1	<6.1	<7.0
and			
2-hour post-glucose load	≥6.7 to <10.0	≥7.8 to <11.1	≥7.8 to <11.1

World Health Organization. Report of a WHO consultation, 1999.

Table 1.3 WHO diagnostic criteria: impaired fasting glucose (IFG)

	Glucose concentration (mmol/l)		
	Whole blood venous	Whole blood capillary	Plasma venous
Impaired fasting glucose			
Fasting	≥5.6 to <6.1	≥5.6 to <6.1	≥6.1 to <7.0
and (if measured)			
2-hour post-glucose load	<6.7	<7.8	<7.8

World Health Organization. Report of a WHO consultation, 1999.

Further reading

Diabetes UK fact sheet May 2000

The Expert Committee on the Diagnosis and classification of diabetes Mellitus 1997. *Diabetes Care* **20**: 1183–1203

Pickup J C, Williams G 2003 *Textbook of Diabetes,* 3rd edn. Oxford: Blackwell Science.

Watkins P J, Amiel S A, Howell S L et al 2003 *Diabetes and its management,* 6th edn. Oxford: Blackwell Publishing

Williams G, Pickup J C 1999 *Handbook of diabetes,* 2nd edn. Oxford: Blackwell Science

World Health Organization 1999 *Report of a WHO consultation.* Geneva

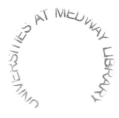

2
Clinical presentation of diabetes mellitus

Type 1 diabetes

The clinical features of type 1 diabetes tend to present more acutely than those of type 2 diabetes.

Young patients typically have a short history (a few days or weeks) of the classic symptoms of:

- thirst, which is often intense;
- polyuria — the passage of large amounts of urine (perhaps several litres per day) due to the osmotic diuresis caused by high glucose and ketone body concentrations in urine;
- rapid weight loss due to the absence of the anabolic actions of insulin and the virtually unopposed actions of glucagon and the counter-regulatory hormones. The effect is increased appetite but also increased dehydration and catabolism of muscle and fat;
- some patients present in the dangerous state of keto-acidosis;
- blurring of vision can also be a presenting symptom due to osmotic disturbances in the crystalline lens;
- sleep is disturbed by nocturia and previously continent children may develop enuresis.

The symptoms of thirst, polyuria and weight loss should always point to a diagnosis of type 1 diabetes mellitus until proven otherwise.

In children these symptoms in combination with a positive urine test for glucose demand immediate referral to a paediatrician.

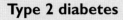
Type 2 diabetes

The presenting features of type 2 diabetes tend to be less acute and dramatic.

They include:

- malaise and fatigue;
- thirst and polyuria;
- blurred vision due to swelling of the crystalline lens;
- infections:
  - thrush vulvo-vaginitis or balanitis;
  - recurrent septic skin infections.

The signs of complications include:

- retinopathy;
- cataract;
- neuropathy;
- myocardial infarction;
- stroke;
- peripheral vascular disease;
- foot ulceration or even gangrene.

In the UK Prospective Diabetes Study (UKPDS), 50% of all newly diagnosed patients with type 2 diabetes had complications at diagnosis. The UKPDS also showed that lowering of glycosylated haemoglobin (HbA1C) levels and tight control of blood pressure reduced the risk of complications (Figs. 2.1–2.3).

A significant number of cases of type 2 diabetes are diagnosed by a positive urine test during a routine medical examination, e.g. for pre-employment or insurance purposes.

In intensively treated patients, HbA1C was 7.0% compared to 7.9% in conventionally treated patients. This 0.9% decrease in HbA1C is associated with a reduction in risk for diabetic complications

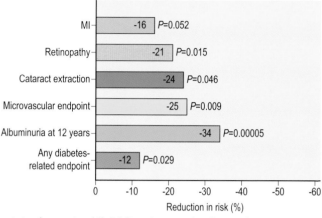

Fig. 2.1 Lowering HbA1C reduces risk of complications.

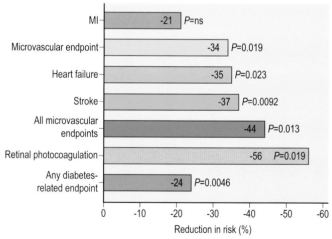

Fig. 2.2 Tight control of BP reduces risk of complications.

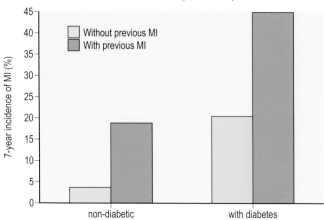

Fig. 2.3 The need to treat cardiovascular risk factors.

3
Type 1 diabetes mellitus

WITHDRAWN FROM UNIVERSITIES AT MEDWAY LIBRARY

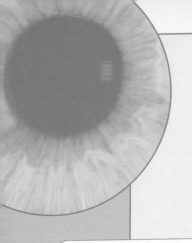

Pathogenesis

In type 1 diabetes there is an auto-immune-mediated selective destruction of the beta cells of the pancreas in genetically susceptible individuals. This results in a very severe deficiency of insulin or even its total absence.

People with type 1 diabetes require insulin for their very survival. There is a breakdown of the glucose homeostasis because of the absence of the glucose-lowering effects of insulin and the unopposed action of glucagon and the counter-regulatory hormones.

A severe deficiency of insulin will impact on carbohydrate, fat and protein metabolism with far reaching consequences (Fig. 3.1).

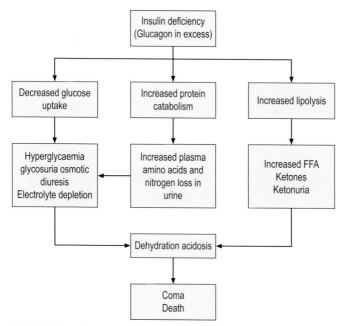

Fig. 3.1   Type 1 summary of insulin deficiency.

Carbohydrate metabolism

Due to the absence of insulin, the blood sugar lowering effect is lost and blood sugar levels rise. In the absence of insulin, there is no inhibition of gluconeogenesis in the liver, and an unopposed glucagon effect on increasing glycogen breakdown to glucose, both of which add to rising blood glucose levels — hyperglycaemia.

The hyperglycaemia is followed by glycosuria because the capacity of the renal tubules to re-absorb glucose is greatly exceeded.

Rising glucose levels increase the osmolarity of the blood, and excretion of the osmotically active glucose molecules involves the loss of large volumes of water, leading to a state of dehydration. This in turn activates the mechanisms in regulating water intake resulting in polydipsia.

In addition to losing water, there is also an appreciable loss of sodium and potassium in the osmotic diuresis caused by the high blood glucose levels.

Although people with type 1 diabetes tend to have enhanced appetite, this only serves to raise blood glucose levels.

While there is an extracellular excess of glucose there is an intracellular glucose deficiency so that cells are robbed of their major source of energy.

The effects of intracellular glucose deficiency

In the absence of glucose, the major source of energy, alternative sources have to be found. This means drawing on reserves of energy in protein and fat stores under the influence of glucagon. Protein and fat are broken down (catabolized) to provide energy. This contributes to the weight loss and wasting which is a clinical feature of type 1 diabetes.

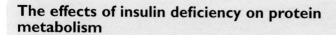

The effects of insulin deficiency on protein metabolism

The inhibitory effect of insulin on protein breakdown (catabolism) is lost. The unopposed action of glucagon increases the rate of protein catabolism and further contributes to the weight loss and wasting seen in type 1 diabetes.

In type 1 diabetes, the net effect of accelerated protein catabolism to produce carbon dioxide, water and glucose under the influence of glucagon is not matched by an increase in protein synthesis because of the deficiency of insulin. The result is a negative nitrogen balance.

The effects of insulin deficiency on fat metabolism

The deficiency of insulin means that the enzyme hormone sensitive lipase is not inhibited. In addition the catabolic effect of glucagon is not opposed by insulin so that the net effect is the release of free fatty acids and plasma levels can double.

Under the influence of insulin, 50% of ingested glucose is normally burned to carbon dioxide and water; 5% converted to glycogen; and 45% converted to fat to be stored in fat deposits. In type 1 diabetes, less than 5% of ingested glucose is converted to fat which further increases blood glucose levels.

Ketosis

As a result of the increased fat catabolism due to insulin deficiency, and the action of glucagon being unopposed, the liver is bombarded with their breakdown products. These are converted in the liver to ketones: acetoacetate and its derivatives acetone and β-hydroxybutyrate, which then enter the circulation in large quantities and are important sources of energy.

However, in untreated type 1 diabetes production exceeds utilization so that a state of ketosis occurs.

Acidosis

Although some of the hydrogen ions liberated from the breakdown of ketones are buffered, a state of acidosis still develops. The resulting low plasma PH stimulates the respiratory centre resulting in the rapid deep respiration known as Kussmaul's breathing.

The loss of water and electrolytes produces a state of dehydration and hypovolaemia and hypotension.

If untreated, the state of dehydration and acidosis can depress consciousness to the point of coma and even death.

Diabetic keto-acidosis is a serious medical emergency requiring urgent fluid and electrolytic replacement and treatment with exogenous insulin.

Insulin

Insulin is synthesized in the B cells of the islets of Langerhans from a single amino acid precursor molecule called proinsulin. This is synthesized from preproinsulin which is cleaved by protease activity to proinsulin. The gene for preproinsulin is located on chromosome 11. Proinsulin is stored in vesicles within the Golgi apparatus of the B cells. From these, secretory granules are matured, which finally break away or bud off, at which time proinsulin is converted to insulin by enzymes and connecting (C) peptide (Fig. 3.2).

The islets of Langerhans secrete at least four peptides with hormonal activity. Two of these, insulin and glucagon, have

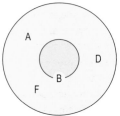

Fig. 3.2 Structure of the islets.

important functions in the metabolism of carbohydrates, proteins and fats.

The third hormone, somatostatin, plays a role in islet cell secretion while the fourth, pancreatic polypeptide, is mainly concerned with gastrointestinal function.

Insulin is anabolic in that it stimulates the storage of glucose, fatty acids and amino acids. Glucagon, on the other hand, is catabolic, mobilizing glucose, fatty acids and amino acids from their stores.

Thus the two hormones are reciprocal in their overall actions and are normally secreted reciprocally.

Insulin excess causes hypoglycaemia (low blood sugar), while insulin deficiency, either absolute or relative, causes diabetes mellitus.

Islets of Langerhans

These are located in the pancreas (Fig. 3.3). In humans they number 250 000–500 500. Each has a copious blood supply which drains directly into the portal vein. The blood flow within the islets flows centrifugally so that the different cells are supplied in a particular order. The islets are made up of four types of cells named A, B, D and F. The blood is supplied B to A to D then F. The structure of the islets is shown diagrammatically in Fig. 3.2.

A single islet is about 0.2 mm in diameter.

The secretions of the islet cells are:

- A (α) cells — glucagon;
- B (β) cells — insulin;
- D (δ) cells — somatostatin;
- F (ϕ) cells — pancreatic polypeptide.

The different cell types can be identified by various techniques including immunostaining techniques and electron microscope appearance of the secretory granules. The B cells are the most common and are located in the core of the islet, while A and F cells are located peripherally. B cells are programmed to synthesize insulin and have a very sophisticated mechanism to regulate its secretion (Fig. 3.3b). The islets are densely innervated with autonomic and peptidergic nerves. Parasympathetic innervation is supplied via the vagus nerve which stimulates insulin release.

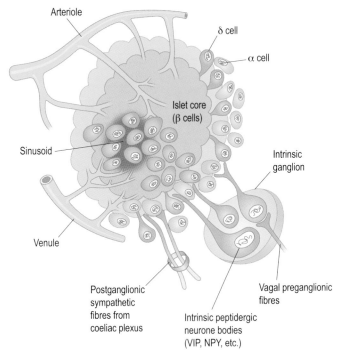

Fig. 3.3a Diagrammatic illustration of the structure of the islets of Langerhans.

Conversely adrenergic sympathetic nerves inhibit insulin and stimulate glucagon secretion. Other nerves that originate in the pancreas contain peptides such as vasoactive intestinal peptide (VIP). This is responsible for the stimulation and release of all islet hormones and neuropeptide Y (NPY) which inhibits insulin secretion. Exactly how all these different neuropeptides all interact is still not fully understood.

The regulation of insulin secretion

The most influential factor in the regulation of insulin secretion is the change in blood glucose concentrations. The responses to

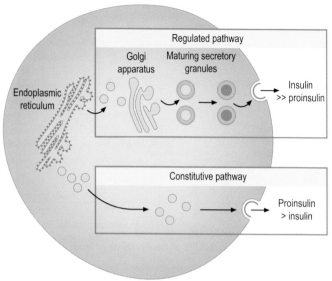

Fig. 3.3b Diagrammatic representation of the intra-cellular production of insulin.

these changes are both sensitive and rapid — usually within 30 seconds of the arrival of a glucose stimulus.

Glucose-stimulated insulin release is biphasic — a rapid first phase lasting some 5–10 minutes followed by a more prolonged second phase which continues for as long as the duration of the stimulus (see Fig. 3.4).

The half-life of insulin in the circulation in humans is about 5 minutes.

The effects of insulin

Insulin's physiological effects are far reaching and comprehensive and affect the metabolism of carbohydrates, fats and proteins. They can conveniently be divided into rapid, intermediate and delayed. These are shown in Box 3.1.

The effects of insulin on adipose tissue, muscle and liver are detailed in Box 3.2.

formation, an alternative source of fuel for the brain when glucose is not available.

Insulin receptors

Cells which are insulin sensitive have a specific insulin receptor on their outer cell surface. Insulin binds to this and then triggers its effects. Not all tissues are insulin sensitive. The brain is the most unresponsive; other non-responsive organs are the intestine and kidney.

Glucose transport

Glucose enters cells by a process of facilitated diffusion, or in the kidneys and intestine, by secondary active transport with sodium. Insulin facilitates glucose entry by increasing the number of glucose transporters in the cell membrane.

Clearly any interference with insulin receptors and/or glucose transport could impair the action on insulin.

Other influences on blood glucose regulation

Insulin is the only hormone that lowers blood glucose concentrations. Corticosteroids, adrenaline, growth hormone and glucagon can all increase blood glucose levels. Thus glucose homeostasis is dependent on striking a right balance between the effects of insulin and the effects of the hormones which raise blood glucose levels.

Type 1 diabetes management

Diet and lifestyle modification are the cornerstones of management in both type 1 and type 2 diabetes.

In type 1 diabetes, dietary recommendations should be matched to a person's overall lifestyle including occupation. For instance, the energy needs of someone doing heavy manual work are much greater than those of a sedentary worker.

The diet must also meet the macro and micro nutritional needs of the individual in order to achieve normoglycaemia and reduce the risk of cardiovascular disease.

It is customary to reduce the intake of saturated fat, to provide no more than 30% of energy requirements and to replace this by mono- and polyunsaturated fats.

Carbohydrates which rapidly raise the blood glucose levels after their ingestion are discouraged and replaced by those with a lower glycaemic index such as whole grain foods, legumes, fruit and nuts.

Fish oils, which are rich in n-3 fatty acids, lower triglyceride levels (which tend to be raised in people with diabetes) so two or three servings of oily fish weekly are beneficial.

Alcohol has a protective effect on cardiovascular disease, if taken in moderate amounts, by raising high density lipoprotein (HDL) cholesterol (the protective cholesterol), decreasing coagulation factors and enhancing insulin sensitivity, so light to moderate drinking should not be discouraged.

Practical food recommendations

- Quench thirst with water or non-sugary drinks.
- Have regular meals.
- Avoid fried and very sugary foods.
- Eat plenty of legumes, whole grain foods or brown rice as part of main meals. They have a low glycaemic index (GI).
- Limit the consumption of starchy foods such as mashed potatoes and white bread.
- Five portions of fruit and vegetables each day.
- For snacks, avoid biscuits or confectionary — use fruit and nuts.
- Limit the intake of red meat, eggs, liver and high fat dairy products. Instead, use lean meats, poultry (without skin) and low fat dairy products.
- Cook and fry with natural vegetable oils.
- Use soft instead of hard margarine.
- Do not over eat.

Smoking

This should be strongly discouraged. It is a major risk factor for cardiovascular disease (CVD) and lung cancer. Stopping smoking is as effective as lowering cholesterol and treating hypertension in reducing CVD.

Exercise

Regular exercise should be encouraged. It improves glycaemic control and lowers long-term morbidity and mortality. Patients should carry measures to combat hypoglycaemia should this occur.

The use of insulin

Type 1 diabetes is a disease of insulin deficiency, and insulin replacement is necessary for survival. Insulin is normally given by a subcutaneous injection.

In non-diabetic people, blood glucose levels are maintained within a fairly narrow range by a combination of endogenous insulin and regulatory hormones.

The current approach to the use of insulin in people with type 1 diabetes is to recreate this physiological state as closely as possible.

To do this there are a plethora of insulin preparations available but basically they can be divided into three types, based on their rapidity and duration of action (see Table 3.1).

Analogue insulins

Analogue insulins have been modified to make them closely resemble naturally occurring human insulin and to make achieving glucose control closely resemble the normal physiological state. The word 'analogue' conveys the meaning of similar to, in this case similar to human insulin, but not an exact replicate. Like human insulins they are genetically engineered. There are rapid

Table 3.1   Some commonly used insulin preparations

	Time of action (hours)			
Insulin class	**Onset**	**Peak**	**Duration**	**Species/ origin**
Short acting				
Monomeric (Lispro, Aspart)	<0.5	0.5–2.5	3.0–4.5	Synthetic
Short-acting soluble	0.3–0.5	1.0–3.0	4.0–8.0	Human Porcine Bovine
Intermediate acting				
Osophane (NPH)	1.0–2.0	4.0–6.0	8.0–12.0	Human Porcine Bovine
Lente	1.0–2.0 1.0–3.0	4.0–8.0 5.0–10.0	8.0–14.0 10.0–24.0	Human Porcine Bovine
Long acting				
Ultra Lente	2.0–3.0 2.0–4.0	4.0–8.0 6.0–12.0	8.0–14.0 12.0–28.0	Human Bovine
Analogues, e.g. (Largine)	0.75–1.5	Peakless	16.0–24.0	Synthetic

and long-acting analogue insulins and there are mixtures of the two. Examples of rapid-acting analogue insulins are:

- Insulin Lispro (Humalog).
- Insulin Aspart (Novo Rapid).
- Insulin Glulisine (Aspiara).

Long-acting analogues include:

- Insulin Glargine (Lantus).
- Insulin Determir (Levemir).

The trade names are given in brackets.

Currently there are three analogue mixtures which are: Humalog Mix 25, Humalog Mix 50 and Novo Mix 30.

The rapid-acting analogue insulins take effect quicker than human or animal short-acting insulins. The latter are usually taken 15–30 minutes before the meal whereas the analogues can be taken just before or during a meal. This is very useful if a person wants to have greater flexibility in choosing meal times.

Long-acting analogues are generally taken once a day at bed time and tend to have a relatively smooth action lasting between 16 and 24 hours.

Both rapid- and long-acting analogue insulins are well suited for basal bolus regimens of insulin delivery (see below). Analogue insulins are not superior to other forms of insulin. Their benefit is that they offer greater flexibility.

Regimes
The two most commonly used insulin regimes are:

- an evening basal bolus (long-acting insulin) with injections of short-acting insulin before each main meal;
- injections of a mixture of short and intermediate insulin, the first before breakfast, the second before the evening meal.

Injection sites
These include the:

- abdomen;
- the outer aspect of the thigh;
- the upper outer buttock.

Injection devices
There are a range of injection devices all designed to make giving the injection easier and less painful.

Side effects of insulin therapy
Insulin is remarkably well tolerated. The commonest side effect is hypoglycaemia.

Other rarer side effects
Lipohypertrophy — fatty bumps at injection sites. These are most likely to occur when insulin is constantly injected into the same site. Rotation of sites helps avoid this.

Some weight gain is inevitable as insulin is primarily an anabolic hormone.

Lipoatrophy — hollowed out areas mainly due to immune responses to impurities in insulin. Rare with newer, more pure insulins.

Glucose monitoring
At the start of insulin therapy, people with diabetes are also taught how to monitor their blood glucose levels.

The blood glucose test is normally prepared from a drop of capillary blood obtained from the side of a fingertip using a modern spring-loaded device.

Tests are normally done before meals and before going to bed. However, if before-meal tests are reasonable but the HbA1C is raised, it is then usual practice to add post-prandial monitoring about 90 minutes after a meal. The frequency of glucose monitoring should be largely determined by the person with diabetes hopefully taking into account professional advice.

Target values for blood glucose levels
These are: 4.0–7.0 m.mols/l before meals and 6.0–9.0 m.mols/l after meals.

Further reading

Al-Delaimy W K, Willett W C, Manson J E et al 2001 Smoking and mortality among women with Type 2 Diabetes. *Diabetes Care* **24**: 2043–2048

Elison L J, Longo M 1992 Glucose transporters. *Annual Review of Medicine* **43**: 377–385

Gamong W F 1999 *Review of medical physiology*, 19th edn. Connecticut, US: Appleton & Lange, p 303–318

Hu F B, Manson J E 2003 Management of diabetes: diet and lifestyle modification. In: Pickup J C, Williams G (eds) *Textbook of diabetes*, 3rd edn. Oxford: Blackwell Science, p 36.1–36.13

Sigal R J, Kenny G P, Koivisto V A 2003 Exercise and diabetes mellitus. In: Pickup J C, Williams G (eds) *Textbook of diabetes*, 3rd edn. Oxford: Blackwell Science, p 37.1–37.19

Watkins P J, Amiel S A, Howell S L et al 2003 *Diabetes and its management*, 6th edn. Oxford: Blackwell Science, p 23–32, 66–78

4
Type 2 diabetes mellitus

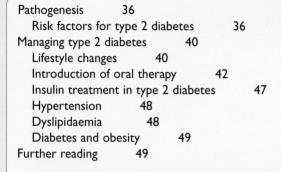

Pathogenesis

The development of type 2 diabetes probably results from an interaction between a genetic predisposition and factors in the environment.

It is a great mistake to think of type 2 diabetes solely in terms of defects in carbohydrate metabolism. It is really a syndrome largely made up of cardiovascular risk factors and about 80% of deaths in people with type 2 diabetes results from cardiovascular causes.

Risk factors for type 2 diabetes

1. Genetic factors
It is much more common to find a positive history in people with type 2 diabetes than it is in type 1. Twin studies have shown a concordance of 60–100% in identical twins and 17% in non-identical twins.

2. Environmental factors
Of these, by far the most common is obesity, as defined by a body mass index (BMI) of >/= 30 kg/m^2. The prevalence of type 2 diabetes is increasing in line with the rising prevalence of obesity, which currently affects 23% of men and 23.5% of women in England.

Not all obese people develop diabetes and not all people with type 2 diabetes are obese but there is clearly a strong association. The prevalence of type 2 diabetes rises in proportion to levels of obesity in the population. A man with a BMI of >35 kg/m^2 has a 40-fold increased risk of developing diabetes.

In females the risk rises above a BMI of 22 with a 5-fold increase at a BMI of 25; a 28-fold increased risk at a BMI of 30; and a 93-fold increased risk at a BMI above 35.

Abdominal obesity (apple-shaped) is more contributory than gluteo-femoral (pear-shaped) obesity, as it is associated with a higher level of insulin resistance and abdominal adipocytes are metabolically more active.

Probably the next most important environmental factors are physical inactivity and inappropriate diet (too high in calories and saturated fat). Both contribute to the development of obesity but regular exercise improves insulin sensitivity and increases the uptake of glucose into muscle tissue. Regular exercise reduces a person's risk of developing type 2 diabetes. Increasing age is associated with a rising risk of diabetes.

3. Fundamental defects in type 2 diabetes

These are insulin resistance and beta cell dysfunction.

Insulin resistance

This is defined as 'the inability of insulin to produce its usual biological effects at concentrations that are effective in normal subjects' (Fig. 4.1). Insulin resistance is in part due to fat deposition within muscle, liver and islet cells which occurs with obesity.

Imbalance of glucose homeostasis While there is a close relationship of obesity to insulin resistance there is also a genetic component. It has been shown that insulin resistance is present in first-degree relatives of people with type 2 diabetes even though they have normoglycaemia. However, this is bought at a price, as their beta cells are having to secrete more insulin leading to a state of hyperinsulinaemia, which is itself a risk factor for cardiovascular disease.

Insulin resistance is important because of its impact on certain key tissues and organs.

Insulin resistance in adipocytes means that insulin's ability to suppress hormone-sensitive lipase (which breaks down fatty tissues to produce non-essential fatty acids (NEFAs)) is diminished. This leads to the release of large amounts of NEFAs into the portal vein and subsequently into the systemic circulation (Fig. 4.2).

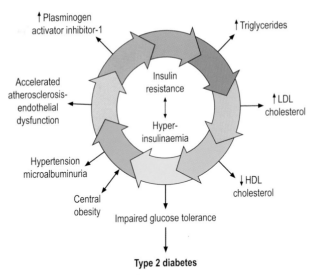

Fig. 4.1 Insulin resistance syndrome.

The portal vein carries blood to the liver and the excess of NEFAs provide fuel for gluconeogenesis, their conversion to blood glucose. The inhibition of this process by insulin has been reduced by the presence of insulin resistance.

When the NEFAs reach skeletal muscle they provide an alternative source of energy to glucose by substrate competition. In addition the uptake of glucose by skeletal muscle, which in health accounts for about 80% of glucose disposal after a meal, is also impaired by post-insulin receptor damage which affects both oxidative glucose disposal and glycogen synthesis.

The higher levels of NEFAs seen in obesity and type 2 diabetes exert a toxic effect on the B cells of the pancreas (Fig. 4.1).

Beta cell failure
The second major defect in type 2 diabetes is beta cell dysfunction and failure.

This is first seen as loss of the first-phase insulin response to a glucose load which in turn causes post-prandial peaks of

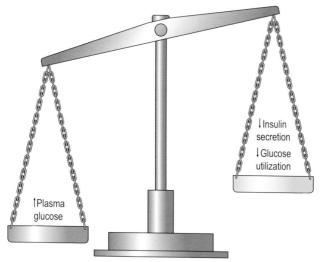

Fig. 4.2 Imbalance of glucose homeostasis.

blood glucose, which are themselves a risk factor for cardiovascular disease.

Damage to the beta cells is caused by the 'toxic' effects of a large number of substances which together have been termed by Matthew Hayden — 'The A-FLIGHT toxicities'. They are:

A   Amylin, which is secreted along with insulin by beta cells.
      Advanced glycosylation end products.
      Anti-oxidant reserve diminished.
F   Free fatty acid toxicity.
L   Lipotoxicity.
I   Insulin.
G   Glucotoxicity.
H   Hypertension toxicity.
      Homocysteine toxicity.
T   Triglyceride toxicity.

These produce progressive damage to the islet cells of the pancreas with a progressive reaction in their ability to produce insulin.

Unlike type 1 diabetes, type 2 diabetes is of insidious onset and this process probably occurs over many years.

The natural history of type 2 diabetes is depicted in Fig. 4.3.

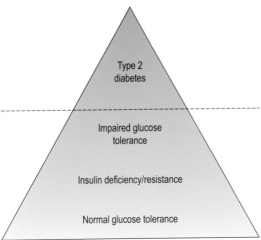

Fig. 4.3
Fig. 4.3
Natural history
of type 2
diabetes.

Managing type 2 diabetes

Treatment principles are summarized in Fig. 4.4 for diabetes
which is a complex metabolic disorder (Fig. 4.5).

Lifestyle changes

These basically involve:

- dietary modification;
- increased physical activity;
- smoking cessation — if a smoker.

Dietary modification

Dietary modification is a key element of managing type 2
diabetes. The diet should aid metabolic control by tackling the
hyperglycaemia and the dyslipidaemia which are features of type 2
diabetes. In addition, as most people with type 2 diabetes are
overweight or obese, it must also contribute to weight loss.

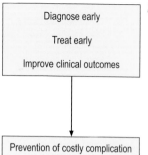

Diagnose early

Treat early

Improve clinical outcomes

Fig. 4.4 Treatment principles.

Prevention of costly complication

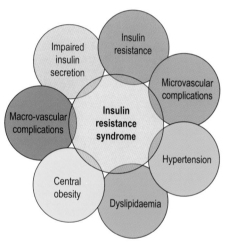

Fig. 4.5 Type 2 diabetes: a complex metabolic disorder.

Thus the diet should:

- be hypocaloric with a deficit of about 600 kcals to normal daily recommendations;
- be low in saturated fat, which should be replaced by mono- and polyunsaturated fat and complex carbohydrates;
- contain complex carbohydrates which are slowly absorbed and less likely to rapidly raise blood sugar levels, which would be the case with simple sugars;
- supply all macro- and micro-nutrients;

mally be low in salt as many people with type 2 diabetes
so have a raised blood pressure;

be individualized taking into account age, occupation, levels of
physical activity and BMI;

- contain five portions of fruit and vegetables daily.

Physical activity

This is particularly beneficial in type 2 diabetes because it:

- increases insulin sensitivity by decreasing insulin resistance;
- lowers blood glucose levels by encouraging the uptake of glucose by muscle tissue;
- raises HDL-C, the 'protective cholesterol';
- aids weight loss and thereafter helps weight maintenance;
- improves physical fitness and overall well-being.

Although the World Health Organization currently recommends 30 minutes of brisk activity daily, nearer 90 minutes are required to make a meaningful contribution to weight loss. However, this can be achieved by adding together shorter periods of physical activity (Figs. 4.6 and 4.7). This could well be easier to fit in a busy lifestyle.

Smoking cessation

Smoking and type 2 diabetes are a lethal combination and patients who smoke should be offered referral to smoking cessation services.

Introduction of oral therapy

Few patients can achieve and sustain adequate control by lifestyle changes for more than a few months. Oral treatment must be considered when:

- usually HbA1C >6.5% and fasting plasma glucose >6.0 mmol/l;
- or (occasionally) if thin and no arterial risk factors. HbA1C >7.5% and fasting plasma glucose = 7.0 mmol/l.

Some options are discussed.

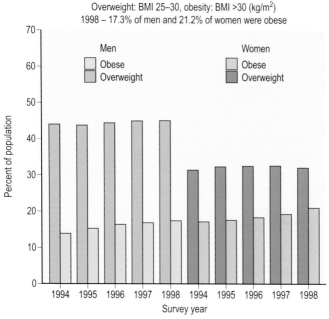

Fig. 4.6 Obesity in the UK population.

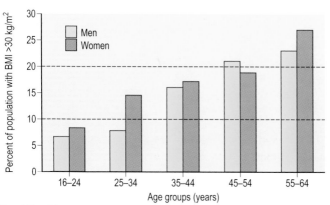

Fig. 4.7 Obesity and increasing age in the UK.

Metformin

This acts by decreasing the production of glucose by the liver (gluconeogenesis) and by decreasing insulin resistance, thereby increasing uptake and utilization of glucose, particularly by skeletal muscle. Metformin reduces plasma glucose levels by 3–4 mmol/l with a larger effect on post-prandial than fasting levels.

In addition it has other beneficial effects:

- does not cause weight gain;
- does not cause hypoglycaemia;
- has a lipid-lowering effect;
- increases fibrinolysis and decreases platelet aggregation;
- the last two points above decrease cardiovascular risk.

Its main side-effects are gastrointestinal and include nausea, vomiting and diarrhoea. These can be minimized by starting with a low dose and increasing slowly, say at weekly intervals, and by taking it with meals.

A rarer side-effect is lactic-acidosis, which is potentially fatal but fortunately rare (3/100 000 cases per year).

The risk can be minimized by avoiding the use of the drug when renal function is impaired (creatinine >160 mmol/l).

Metformin is the drug of choice in people with type 2 diabetes who are overweight or obese and with no contraindications. It can be used in combination with a sulphonylurea and as an adjunct to insulin therapy. It is contraindicated in:

- renal failure;
- severe cardiac failure;
- hepatic failure;
- alcohol abuse.

Thiazolinediones (glitazones)

These represent a significant breakthrough in the treatment of type 2 diabetes because they effectively tackle one of its major causes — insulin resistance.

As a result they:

- decrease hepatic gluconeogenesis and thereby hepatic glucose output;

- decrease the release of non-sterified fatty acids from adipocytes;
- increase the uptake of glucose and utilization of glucose by muscle;
- decrease fasting glycaemia by 2.3 mmol/l and decrease HbA1C.

The main side effects are:

- weight gain but this consists of subcutaneous and not visceral fat;
- fluid retention and a mild dilutional anaemia.

They are contra-indicated in heart failure and hepatic failure. The first glitazone, troglitazone, had to be withdrawn because of liver damage but this does not seem to be a problem with the two currently available drugs, pioglitazone and rosiglitazone. Nevertheless, it is recommended that liver function tests should be performed every 2 months in the first year of treatment and periodically thereafter.

The glitazones are currently used as part of combination treatment in people with type 2 diabetes who are not achieving adequate control with monotherapy.

Thus they can be added to a sulphonylurea if metformin is contra-indicated or not tolerated, or added to metformin in obese subjects where further weight gain is not desirable.

Insulin secretagogues
The most commonly used drugs in the groups are the sulphonylureas.

Sulphonylureas (SUs)
These are a group of drugs which stimulate the beta cells to produce insulin. All are largely similar in efficiency but they vary in the duration of action. They tend to lower plasma insulin levels by about 3–4 mmol/l and are more effective in newly diagnosed patients with a reasonable level of beta cell activity still present.

Side-effects

- Probably the most important is hypoglycaemia. It is less likely with shorter acting preparations which are the preferred choice in clinical practice.
- Weight gain (1–2 kg on average).

In fact they are remarkably well tolerated. SUs are the first choice of drug in lean people with type 2 diabetes but can be added to metformin. Examples are tolbutamide, glibenclamide, gliclazide, glipizide, gliquidone and glimeprimide.

Meglitinides

These are rapid- and short-acting secretagogues. Because of their rapid action, they can be taken just before meals. This rapid action helps prevent post-prandial glucose peaks which are thought to be a cardiovascular risk factor.

They are generally regarded as having a fairly low risk of causing hypoglycaemia. Two drugs are currently available: repaglinide and nateglinide.

Repaglinide can be used as monotherapy or in combination with metformin or a glitazone. Nateglinide is used in combination with metformin.

They tend to lower HbA1C by 1–2% and post-prandial glycaemia by 1.4 mmol/l when used alone. In combination they can lower HbA1C by an additional 0.5–1.5% and post-prandial glycaemia by an additional 1–3 mmol/l.

Glucosidase inhibitors (acarbose)

They act by inhibiting the enzymes which break down disaccharides in the intestinal brush border. In doing so, they delay absorption.

They can lower blood glucose levels by 1–2 mmol/l. When taken with a high carbohydrate diet, the malabsorption which they cause leads to bloating, flatulence and diarrhoea.

While trials suggest that they can be as effective as metformin when added to a sulphonylurea, these side effects limit their use.

Insulin treatment in type 2 diabetes

Type 2 diabetes is a progressive disease. Sulphonylureas, meglitinides, metformin and thiazolidinediones are only effective when there is residual beta cell activity.

However, as the disease progresses, more and more beta cells fail and often a time is reached when even combination therapy cannot achieve the targets for adequate control and HbA1C levels less than 8%. At this stage treatment with insulin should be offered.

In type 2 diabetes, insulin can be used in a number of ways. Three examples are described:

1. Patients poorly controlled on combination therapy but still having some beta cells Secretary reserve can be given a single injection of an intermediate-acting insulin at night. The dose will depend on the level of hyperglycaemia and the body weight but a typical starting dose would be 6–10 units, increasing until 4–6 mmols/l fasting plasma glucose.
Oral combination therapy is continued. Such a regime is usually well tolerated. Sometimes the sulphonylurea is withdrawn, as a combination of sulphonylureas and insulin can exacerbate weight gain, but the metformin is continued to exploit the insulin-sensitizing effects.
If control deteriorates, a second morning injection can be added.
2. Tablet treatment can be withdrawn and substituted by twice-daily injection of an intermediate insulin or twice-daily injections of a combination of a short- and an intermediate-acting insulin.
3. A basal bolus regime. This normally consists of an evening injection of an intermediate-acting insulin at night with an injection of a rapidly acting insulin before the three main meals.

Type 2 diabetes is a complex, metabolic disorder. Many people with type 2 diabetes are at increased risk of cardiovascular disease because they also have hypertension, dyslipidaemia and

a pro-coagulant state, all of which should normally be
aggressively treated.

Hypertension

This commonly requires the use of two or three drugs. Blood
pressure drugs used are:

- ACE inhibitors;
- calcium channel blockers;
- beta-blockers;
- thiazide diuretics;
- alpha blockers;
- angiotensin-II receptor blockers (AT-II blocker).

Whatever combination is used it should be matched to the
cardiovascular risk profile of the individual patient.

If microalbuminuria is present an ACE inhibitor or AT-II
blocker would normally be first choice in a patient with
type 2 diabetes.

Dyslipidaemia

This is commonly seen as:

- reduced HDL cholesterol — the protective cholesterol;
- raised triglycerides; and
- small dense LDL cholesterol.

Such a picture is a major risk factor for cardiovascular disease.
Although dietary manipulation can produce some improvement,
drugs are usually needed. Those used tend to be the drugs of
the statin groups, e.g. simvastatin, pravastatin, atorvastatin or
rosuvastatin, or a member of the fibrate groups, e.g. bezafibrate
or fenofibrate.

Choice of drug is made by a consideration of the degree of
lipid abnormality and the patient's risk profile. Sometimes
combination therapy is required.

Diabetes and obesity

Obesity is a major risk factor for type 2 diabetes (Figs. 4.6 and 4.7) and about 85% of people with diabetes are significantly overweight or obese. Losing weight improves control of diabetes and has a favourable effect on cardiovascular risk factors. In fact, achieving a 10% weight loss, significantly reduces blood glucose and blood pressure and improves the dyslipidaemia of diabetes as well as having a beneficial effect on the pro-coagulant state.

All people find achieving and sustaining weight loss difficult but this is particularly applicable to people with type 2 diabetes.

Given the risk profile of people with type 2 diabetes and the known benefits of weight loss, the use of drugs to aid weight loss would appear to be justified.

Two drugs, Orlistat and Sibutramine, are currently available and the use of them is backed by a considerable body of research evidence.

Further reading

Bailey G G, Fiefer M D 2004 *Therapies for diabetes*. London: Sherborne Gibbs, p 51

Chan J M, Rimm E B, Colditz G A et al 1994 Obesity, fat distribution and weight gain as risk factors for clinical diabetes in men. *Diabetes Care* **17**: 961–969

Colditz G A, Willett W C, Ronitzky A et al 1995 Weight gain as a risk factor for clinical diabetes mellitus in women. *Annals of Internal Medicine* **122**: 481–486

The Health Survey for England 2003 Department of Health. London

English P, Williams G 2001 *Type 2 diabetes*. London: Martin Dunitz, p 15, 82

Evans D J, Murray R, Kissebah A H 1984 Relationships between skeletal muscle insulin resistance, insulin mediated glucose disposal and insulin binding effects of obesity and body fat topography. *Journal of Clinical Investigation* **74**: 1515–1525

Fiver N, Bloom S R 2000 Sibutramine is effective for weight loss and diabetic control in obesity with type 2 diabetes: a randomised, double blind, placebo controlled study. *Diabetes, Obesity and Metabolism* **2**: 105–112

Fuchtenbusch M, Standl E, Schatz H 2000 Clinical efficiency of new thiazolidinediones and glinides in the treatment of type 2 diabetes mellitus. *Experimental and Clinical Endocrinology & Diabetes* **108**: 151–163

Hayden M 2002 Islet amyloid metabolite syndrome and the natural progressive history of type 2 diabetes mellitus. J. *Pancreas (JOP)* (online) **3(5)**: 126–138

Hollander P A, Elbein S C, Hirsch I B et al 1998 Role of orlistat in the treatment of obese patients with type 2 diabetes. *Diabetes Care* **21**: 1288–1294

Kaprio J, Tuomilehto J, Kookenvuo M et al 1992 Concordance of type 1 and type 2 diabetes mellitus in a population based cohort of twins in Finland. *Diabetologia* **35**: 1060–1067

Khan C R 1994 Insulin action diabetes. *Diabetes* **43**: 1066–1084

Landgraf R, Bilo H J, Muller P G 1999 A comparison of repaglinide and glibenclamide in the treatment of type 2 diabetic patients previously treated with sulphonylureas. *European Journal of Clinical Pharmacology* **55**: 165–171

Merman B, Selby J C, King M C et al 1987 Concordance for type 2 diabetes in male twins. *Diabetologia* **30**: 763–768

Nolan J J, Jones P, Patwardhan R et al 2000 Rosiglitazone taken once daily provides effective glycaemia control in patients with type 2 diabetes mellitus. *Diabetic Medicine* **17**: 287–294

Reisen E, Abel E, Modan M et al 1978 The effect of weight loss without salt restriction in blood pressure on overweight hypertensive patients. *New England Journal of Medicine* **298**: 1–6

Wielins B, Ruge D 1999 Comparison of acarbose and metformin in patients with type 2 diabetes insufficiently controlled with diet and sulphonylureas; a randomised, placebo controlled study. *Diabetic Medicine* **16**: 755–761

Wing R R, Koeske R, Epstein L H et al 1987 Long term effects of modest weight loss in type 2 diabetic patients. *Archives of Internal Medicine* **147**: 1749–1753

Yki-Jarvien H, Kauppila M, Kujansau E et al 1992 Comparison of insulin regimes in patients with non-insulin dependent diabetes. *New England Journal of Medicine* **231**: 253–260

5
Acute and chronic complications of diabetes mellitus and living with the disease

Acute complications

Acute complications include:

1. Ketoacidosis

This has previously been mentioned. It comprises a triad of abnormalities:

- hyperglycaemia;
- ketosis;
- acidosis.

All of these are required for making the diagnosis of ketoacidosis.

Diabetic ketoacidosis is the presenting feature in about 25% of newly diagnosed cases.

Other causes are:

- severe infection;
- inappropriate professional advice to stop insulin in a patient who is anorectic or vomiting;
- patient deliberately withholding insulin.

As a complication it is mainly associated with type 1 diabetes but can occur in a patient with type 2 diabetes when subjected to the stress of myocardial infarction or a very severe infection.

Diabetic ketoacidosis is a serious medical emergency requiring urgent hospital admission for treatment with insulin and intra-venous fluid replacement.

2. Hypoglycaemia

The word literally means 'low glucose in the blood'. Although mainly found as a complication of insulin therapy, it can occur in people with type 2 diabetes treated with insulin secretagogues. A rare cause is an insulin-secreting tumour in the pancreas.

The symptoms and signs of hypoglycaemia can be largely classified as autonomic or neuroglycopenic and are set out in Tables 5.1 and 5.2.

In children there are additional manifestations such as:

- headache;
- aggression;

Table 5.1   Presentation of acute hypoglycaemia

	Symptoms	
Autonomic	**Neuroglycopenic**	**Other**
Sweating	Loss of concentration	Hunger
Shakiness	Drowsiness	Blurred vision
Feeling anxious	Dizziness	Weakness
Nausea		
Pounding heart		

Table 5.2   Signs of acute hypoglycaemia

Pallor	Confusion
Tremor	Irritability
Sweating	Slurred speech
Tachycardia	Lethargy
	Coma
	Seizure
	Hemiparesis

- foolishness;
- naughtiness;
- irritability;
- sadness;
- nightmares;
- nausea;
- convulsions.

Hypoglycaemia is caused by a combination of two factors:

1. elevation of circulating insulin levels beyond the normal therapeutic range;
2. an inadequate counter-regulatory response.

Most patients on insulin recognize the early symptoms and signs and take appropriate action, e.g. three glucose tablets, Lucozade (100–150 mls), fresh orange juice or other non-diet drinks.

However, severe hypoglycaemia can occur in people who have had type 1 diabetes for several years who, due to autonomic nerve damage, lose their hypoglycaemic awareness. This can cause severe problems.

The management of hypoglycaemia, both mild and severe, is outlined in Table 5.3.

Severe complications

First, intra-muscular glucagon 1 mgm, is usually effective in 10 minutes, then longer acting carbohydrate, e.g. digestive biscuit, banana or intravenous glucose 75 mls of 20% glucose solution.

The chronic complications are (Figs. 5.1 and 5.2):

- retinopathy — the most common cause of blindness in people of working age. Diabetic eye disease is dealt with in detail in the following chapters;
- nephropathy — 16% of all new patients needing renal replacement therapy have diabetes;
- erectile dysfunction — may affect up to 50% of men with long-standing diabetes;

Table 5.3   Treatment of hypoglycaemia

Mild	Lucozade	100–150 mls
	Fruit Juice	150–200 mls
	Lemonade	150–200 mls
	Coca-Cola	150–200 mls
	(non-diet)	
	Hypostop glucose gel	

Repeat after 5 minutes if no improvement. Then consume one slice of bread if meal within 1 hour or two slices of bread if not for 2 hours or if at night.

Check blood glucose after 30 minutes to ensure recovery i.e. >4 m.mol/l.

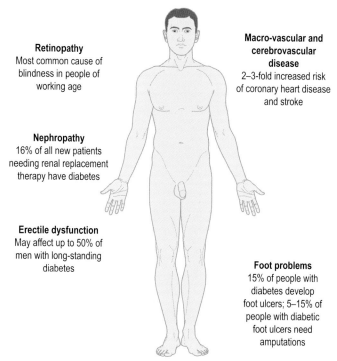

Retinopathy
Most common cause of blindness in people of working age

Nephropathy
16% of all new patients needing renal replacement therapy have diabetes

Erectile dysfunction
May affect up to 50% of men with long-standing diabetes

Macro-vascular and cerebrovascular disease
2–3-fold increased risk of coronary heart disease and stroke

Foot problems
15% of people with diabetes develop foot ulcers; 5–15% of people with diabetic foot ulcers need amputations

Fig. 5.1 Chronic complications of diabetes.

- macro-vascular and cerebrovascular disease — 2–3-fold increased risk of coronary heart disease and stroke;
- foot ulcers — 15% of people with diabetes develop foot ulcers; 5–15% of people with diabetic foot ulcers need amputation.

Living with diabetes mellitus

Diabetes is a lifelong condition associated with a number of serious complications.

It has a major impact on the lives of those who have it and has repercussions for their families.

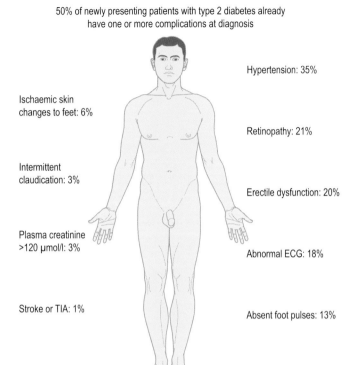

50% of newly presenting patients with type 2 diabetes already have one or more complications at diagnosis

Hypertension: 35%

Ischaemic skin changes to feet: 6%

Retinopathy: 21%

Intermittent claudication: 3%

Erectile dysfunction: 20%

Plasma creatinine >120 µmol/l: 3%

Abnormal ECG: 18%

Stroke or TIA: 1%

Absent foot pulses: 13%

Myocardial infarction: 1%

Fig. 5.2 Complications at diagnosis in the UKPDS.

A life dominated by the need to follow dietary advice, eat at regular times, swallow increasing amounts of medication or to regularly self-inject can hardly be described as normal.

Diabetes impacts on a person's life in a great many ways and puts people at increased risk of:

- cardiovascular disease;
- renal disease;
- eye disease;
- premature mortality.

Little wonder then that depressive illness is three times more common in people with diabetes.

However, it has to be said that the majority of people with diabetes adapt to its demands remarkably well and lead full and active lives, given appropriate advice and support, but not without considerable personal effort.

Employment

Insulin-treated people with diabetes cannot enter:

- the armed forces;
- the fire services;
- the merchant navy;
- the police (although this is being reviewed).

They cannot serve as pilots or hold licences for heavy goods and passenger-carrying vehicles. Shift work for people on insulin injections can pose many problems.

Leisure activities

Physically active sports pose problems for people treated with insulin and requires careful management of dosage and dietary intake, usually involving multiple blood tests.

Driving

People treated with tablets and/or insulin must inform the DVLA at Swansea. If they are not suffering from blackouts they can hold a Group 1 (Category B) driving licence.

Travel

Long haul travel poses particular problems. Dietary arrangements can be upset and injection regimes have to be modified. Injection times are normally lengthened by 2–3 hours when flying west and shortened by 2–3 hours when flying east. But blood glucose levels have to be closely monitored and this usually means extra blood tests. Basal bolus regimes are particularly suited to long haul flights.

Insurance

A diagnosis of diabetes normally carries with it extra loading for life insurance, sickness and holiday insurance.

Further reading

Amiel S A 1998 Hypoglycaemia associated syndrome. The Ernst Frederich Pfeiffer Memorial Lecture. *Acta Diabetologica* **35**: 226–231

Ross L A, McGrimmon R J, Friet B M et al 1998 Hypoglycaemia symptoms reported in children with Type 1 diabetes mellitus and by their parents. *Diabetic Medicine* **15**: 836–843

Watkins P J, Amiel S A, Howell S L et al 2003 *Diabetes and its management*, 6th edn. Oxford: Blackwell Publishing, p 89

Williams G, Pickup J C 2005 *Hand book of diabetes*, 3rd edn. Oxford: Blackwell Publishing

6
Pathophysiology of diabetic retinopathy

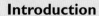

Introduction

Diabetic retinopathy (DR) is the main cause of blindness in the working age group in the UK and most other developed countries. The overall prevalence of diabetic retinopathy varies in different populations but diabetic retinopathy is the major blinding ocular complication of diabetes. The increasing number of individuals with diabetes worldwide suggests that DR and diabetic maculopathy (DM) will continue to be major contributors to vision loss and associated functional impairment for years to come. DR is a potentially visually devastating complication of chronic hyperglycaemia and other associated systemic abnormalities. Advanced stages of DR are characterized by the growth of abnormal retinal blood vessels secondary to ischaemia. These blood vessels grow in an attempt to supply oxygenated blood to the hypoxic retina. At any time during the progression of DR, patients with diabetes can also develop DM, which involves retinal thickening in the macular area. DM occurs after breakdown of the blood-retinal barrier because of leakage of dilated hyperpermeable capillaries and microaneurysms.

Numerous large, prospective randomized clinical trials have delineated the current standard prevention and treatment protocols including intensive glycaemic and blood pressure control and laser photocoagulation for neovascularization and clinically significant macula oedema (see Chapter 8).

The exact mechanisms by which elevated glucose initiates the vascular disruption in retinopathy remain poorly defined, and, not surprisingly, several pathways have been implicated. The vascular disruptions of DR and DM are characterized by abnormal vascular flow, disruptions in permeability, and/or closure or non-perfusion of capillaries. Microvascular leakage and microvascular occlusion are the two main pathological processes responsible for development of the sight-threatening consequences of DR. The structural abnormalities that develop within the retinal capillary wall that lead to these processes include the following (Fig. 6.1):

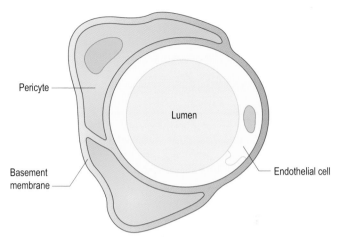

Fig. 6.1 Structure of a retinal capillary.

- pericyte loss;
- loss of endothelial cells;
- basement membrane thickening;
- endothelial cell dysfunction.

Increased retinal vascular permeability results in haemorrhages, exudates and retinal oedema (Fig. 6.2).

Development of microangiopathic changes in diabetic retinopathy

The mechanism of development of microangiopathy is not fully understood, but relates to a combination of changes in ultrastructural, biochemical and haemostatic processes. These include capillary basement membrane thickening (CBMT), non-enzymatic glycosylation, possibly increased free radical activity, increased flux through the polyol pathway and haemostatic abnormalities. The central feature is hyperglycaemia, which is directly linked to the above changes and ultimately causes tissue ischaemia. Many studies have demonstrated that

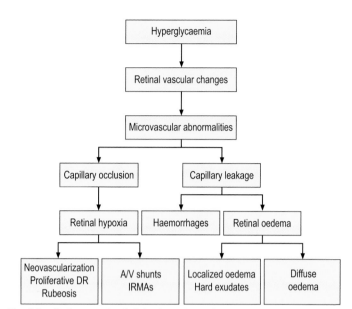

Fig. 6.2 Pathogenesis of diabetic retinopathy.

chronic hyperglycaemia, as well as hyperlipidaemia and hypertension, contribute to the pathogenesis of DR.

Capillary basement membrane thickening (CBMT)

Endothelial cells are responsible for maintaining the blood-retinal barrier, and damage to them results in increased vascular permeability. The histological hallmark of microangiopathy is CBMT. Thickening of the capillary basement membrane and increased deposition of extracellular matrix components may contribute to the development of abnormal retinal haemodynamics, including abnormal auto-regulation of retinal blood flow.

The exact mechanism of thickening and leakiness of the basement membrane appears to involve several biochemical mechanisms and is still not fully understood. The major structural element involved in CBMT is type IV collagen as well as heparin sulphate, an important proteoglycan, together with laminin and fibronectin. Heparin sulphate, produced by the endothelial cells, is highly negatively charged and creates a regular lattice structure of anionic sites that hinders the filtration of negatively charged proteins such as albumin. In diabetes there appears to be impaired synthesis of proteoglycans and an increase in hydroxylysine and its glycosidally linked disaccharide units. Such alterations lead to abnormal packing of the peptide chains which produces excessive leakiness of the membrane. This in part explains the development of e.g. microalbuminuria seen in diabetics.

There is also evidence that retinal leukostasis may play a significant role in the pathogenesis of DR. Leukocytes (white blood cells) possess large cell volumes, high cytoplasmic rigidity, a natural tendency to adhere to the vascular endothelium, and a capacity to generate toxic superoxide radicals and proteolytic enzymes. In diabetes, there is increased retinal leukostasis, which affects retinal endothelial function, retinal perfusion, angiogenesis, and vascular permeability. In particular, leukocytes in diabetes are less deformable, a higher proportion are activated, and they may be involved in capillary non-perfusion, endothelial cell damage, and vascular leakage in the retinal microcirculation. Capillary occlusions, capillary dropout or degeneration associated with leukocytes in the diabetic retina are now thought to be common.

Formation of non-enzymatic glycation products

Another consequence of hyperglycaemia is the formation of modified proteins known as glycation products (Box 6.1). Carbohydrates interact with protein side chains in a

> ### Box 6.1   Non-enzymatic glycosylation of long-lived tissue protein to produce AGEs
>
> Glucose + NH2 + protein $\leftrightarrows$ Schiff base (aldimine) $\leftrightarrows$ Amadori product $\rceil$
>
> Glucose-derived cross linked Advanced glycosylation end-products (AGEs)

non-enzymatic fashion to form Amadori products, and these may subsequently form advanced glycosylation end-products (AGEs), particularly where there is a high glucose concentration.

These products are formed non-enzymatically via a series of intermediate steps. An example is the production of glycosylated haemoglobin (as measured by the HbA1C blood test).

Such products then undergo a series of changes resulting in AGEs. AGEs are resistant to degradation and continue to accumulate indefinitely on long-lived proteins. These may therefore be responsible for the production of CBMT. AGEs may affect such functions as enzyme activity, binding of regulatory molecules, and susceptibility of proteins to proteolysis.

The chronic interaction of these products with at least one specific cell surface receptor for AGEs (AGE-specific receptor) may perpetuate a pro-inflammatory signalling process and a pro-atherosclerotic state in vascular tissues. AGE formation within the endothelial cell basement membrane inactivates endothelial-derived nitric oxide, which acts on peri-vascular smooth muscle causing vasodilation. This may result in impaired blood flow. Several cells, including vascular endothelial cells, possess receptors for AGEs. Binding of AGEs to endothelial receptors causes changes in vascular permeability and favours thrombosis at the endothelial cell surface.

Free radical activity

Free radicals are violently reactive chemicals capable of oxidation of protein amino acid residues as well as lipid peroxidation.

Free radicals are produced continuously during many metabolic processes and are rapidly eliminated by anti-oxidants such as reduced glutathione (GSH) and vitamins C and E. Diabetic patients however have a lower concentration of GSH as well as vitamins C and E. The reduction in anti-oxidant reserve in diabetic patients may be due to competition for nicotinamide adenine dinucleotide phosphate-oxidase (NADPH). This is a co-factor required to re-cycle the oxidized free-radical scavengers back to the effective form (redox cycling). NADPH is produced by the hexose monophosphate shunt and one source of competition from NADHP comes from the polyol pathway. Excess free radicals may be produced either from protein glycation or because of inefficient elimination by reduced anti-oxidants, possibly secondary to NADPH utilization and defective redox cycling.

The polyol pathway

The polyol pathway converts hexose sugars such as glucose into sugar alcohols (polyols). For example glucose can be converted into sorbitol via the action of the enzyme aldose reductase. Aldose reductase is the rate-limiting enzyme for this pathway. Under normal conditions glucose is metabolized via the hexokinase pathway. In the presence of hyperglycaemia high glucose levels saturate the hexokinase pathway and glucose is then metabolized by the polyol pathway. This then has a knock-on effect for other metabolic processes. Increased aldose reductase activity and accumulation of sorbitol have been found in diabetic animal models. As sorbitol does not easily dissolve across cell membranes this increases cellular osmolarity, ultimately leading to cell damage. Increased polyol pathway activity also alters the redox state of the pyridine nucleotides NADP+ and NAD+, thus reducing their concentrations. Since these are important factors in many enzyme-catalysed reactions, many other metabolic pathways may be also affected. The decreased concentration of these cofactors leads to decreased synthesis of reduced gluta-thione, nictric oxide, myoinositol and taurine. Myoinositol is particularly required for the normal function of nerves. Sorbitol may also glycate nitrogens on proteins, such as collagen, producing AGE products.

Protein kinase C activity

Protein kinases are enzymes that modify other proteins by chemically adding phosphate groups to them (phosphorylation). Hyperglycaemia is associated with increased cellular protein kinase C activity in cultured endothelial cells, resulting from enhanced synthesis of diacylglycerol from glucose. Protein kinase C is involved in signal transduction of responses to hormones, growth factors and neurotransmitters. It can affect growth rate, DNA synthesis, hormone receptor turnover and contraction in vascular smooth muscle cells. Protein kinase C activity may have a role in the development of microangiopathy in relation to hyperglycaemia (Fig. 6.3).

Abnormalities in haemostasis

In patients with early DR the likelihood of micro-thrombus formation is enhanced because of an increase of factor VIII, which is produced by the endothelial cells. Another substance called prostacyclin (PGI_2), which is normally produced in endothelial cells, has a strong vasodilator effect that can reduce platelet aggregation and adherence to the cell wall. In diabetic patients production of PGI_2 is reduced. Another substance involved in thrombosis that is in lower concentrations in diabetics is plasminogen activator. This converts plasminogen to plasmin which then promotes fibrinolysis.

Platelet function in diabetes is also abnormal. Thromboxane A_2 which is released from platelets is increased in diabetics (as with many vascular conditions). This produces significant vasoconstriction and also causes platelet aggregation. This combination of factors leads to micro-thrombus formation and small vessel occlusion.

Retinal leukostasis

There is evidence that retinal leukostasis may also play an important role in the pathogenesis of DR. In diabetes there is increased retinal leukostasis, which affects retinal endothelial function, retinal perfusion, angiogenesis and vascular permeability. Leukocytes possess very large cell volume, high cytoplasmic rigidity, and a natural tendency to adhere to the vascular endothelium via cellular adhesion molecules such as intercellular adhesion

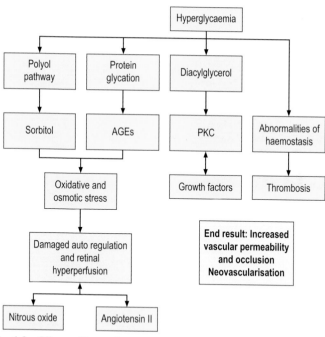

Fig. 6.3 Effects of hyperglycaemia.

molecule-1 (ICAM-1) and beta-integrins on the leukocytes. Other molecules also thought to be involved in this process include: vascular cell adhesion molecules, fibronectin and osteopontin. Furthermore, they are thought to generate toxic superoxide radicals and proteolytic enzymes. In diabetics leukocytes are less deformable, with a relatively high proportion in an activated state, and these factors contribute to capillary non-perfusion, endothelial cell damage and vascular leakage in the retinal microcirculation.

Neovascularisation

As a result of retinal occluded capillaries, retinal ischaemia stimulates a pathologic neovascularization mediated by angiogenic factors, such as vascular endothelial growth factor (VEGF), which ultimately gives rise to proliferative retinopathy.

The exact pathogenesis of retinal neovascularization is not fully understood, although there have been some significant advances in our understanding of this condition in recent years.

It is thought that systemic activation of leucocytes, particularly monocytes, leads to capillary closure through increased adhesiveness of the leucocytes to the damaged endothelial cell surface of the capillary walls. Activated macrophages in the tissues, probably derived from a pool of circulating cells and from a resident microglial population, provide a rich source of growth factors and other molecules such as matrix-modifying enzymes which lead ultimately to an angiogenic response surrounding healthy endothelial cells. It is thought that, for example, heparin-binding growth factors, transforming growth factors and VEGF, which have all been identified in in vitro angiogenetic studies, all may play a part.

Hyperglycaemia (Fig. 6.4) with subsequent protein kinase C activation and release of VEGF are important triggers to the development of retinopathy. VEGF is a potent pro-angiogenic and permeability factor that causes new vessel growth and vascular leakage and is 50 000 times more potent than histamine in producing vascular leakage. It is elevated even in background

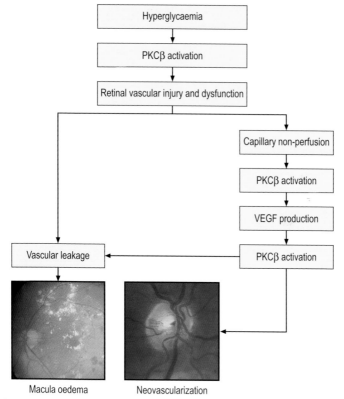

Fig. 6.4 Hyperglycaemia and protein kinase C activation.

DR, is associated with increased vascular permeability, increases with disease severity and is detectable in the vitreous and aqueous once neovascularization has developed. The production of VEGF is induced by hypoxia.

Conclusion

Understanding the diabetes-induced mechanisms that contribute to pericyte loss, endothelial cell proliferation, neovascularization and alterations in basement membrane structure is very important in the design of pharmacological therapeutic strategies to treat and prevent the early diabetes-related microvascular changes.

Further reading

Barnett A H 1993 Origin of the microangiopathic changes in diabetes. *Eye* **7**: 218–222

Garner A 1993 Histopathology of diabetic retinopathy in man. Eye 7:250–253

Kampik A, Ulbig M 1990 Diabetic retinopathy. *Current Opinion in Ophthalmology* **1**: 161–166

Lawrenson J G 2000 Histopathology and pathogenesis of diabetic retinopathy. In: Rudnicka A R, Birch J (eds) *Diabetic eye disease: identification and management.* Oxford: Butterworth-Heinemann

Little H L, Sachs A H 1977 Role of abnormal blood rheology in the pathogenesis of diabetic retinopathy. *Transactions of the American Academy of Ophthalmology* **83**: 522–561

Miyamato K, Ogura Y 1999 Pathogenetic potential of leukocytes in diabetic retinopathy. *Seminars in Ophthalmology* **14**: 233–239

Stanga P E, Boyd S R, Hamilton A M P 1999 Ocular manifestations of diabetes mellitus. *Current Opinion in Ophthalmology* **10**: 483–489

Zata R, Brenner B M 1986 Pathogenesis of diabetic microangiopathy. *American Journal of Medicine* **80**: 443–453

7
Clinical features of diabetic retinopathy

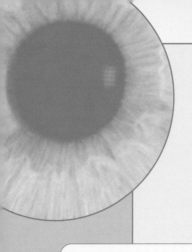

Introduction

Diabetic retinopathy (DR) was first described in 1855 by Jaeger just a few years after the invention of the ophthalmoscope. DR is a chronic progressive sight-threatening disease of the retinal microvasculature associated with prolonged hyperglycaemia and other conditions linked to diabetes mellitus such as hypertension.

DR is a potentially blinding disease in which the threat to sight comes from two main causes. These are damage to the macula (i.e. diabetic maculopathy (DM)) causing reduced visual acuity and development of new vessels leading ultimately to intraocular haemorrhage and tractional retinal detachment causing blindness.

Prevalence of diabetic retinopathy (DR)

DR is the most frequent cause of new cases of blindness among adults aged 24–74 years. Up to 21% of patients with type 2 diabetes have retinopathy at the time of diagnosis of diabetes and most develop some degree of retinopathy over time. The United Kingdom Prospective Diabetes Study (UKPDS) found a higher prevalence of DR in men compared with women (35% and 39%, respectively) in newly diagnosed type 2 diabetics. During the first two decades of disease, nearly all patients with type 1 diabetes and over 60% of patients with type 2 diabetes develop DR. Generally, the prevalence of retinopathy at diagnosis of type 1 diabetes is relatively low i.e. between 0% and 3%.

Collated data from a number of recent epidemiological surveys have estimated that of the approximately 10.2 million Americans over the age of 40 years with diabetes, a total of 40.3% have DR and 8.2% have sight-threatening retinopathy. Also it is estimated that among type 1 diabetics, 75–82% have some degree of DR and up to 32% of these patients have DR which is sight threatening.

More recent UK prevalence studies suggest that improvements in treatment of diabetes have led to lower rates of retinopathy, particularly of the sight-threatening type.

Pre-clinical retinopathy and histopathology

One of the earliest reported features of diabetic pre-retinopathy has been the presence of dilated retinal veins. This is extremely difficult to assess and its importance in clinical management is somewhat dubious.

The earliest clinically visible changes that develop are microaneurysms usually temporal to the fovea and representing mild NPDR. They can be classified into two distinct types:

- **Saccular** — sac-like extensions presumed to evolve from weak points in the capillary wall and abetted by intra-luminal pressure. Reduced structural support from pericytes has been suggested as a contributory factor to their formation. An active cellular response, possibly as a result of a reduced inhibitory action by pericytes, has been proposed as a model for microaneurysm formation. In this case there would be an active budding of the cells of the cell wall.
- **Loop** — originate as kinks in a capillary, these appear to be uncommon in non-diabetics in contrast to saccular microaneurysms which are common in many vascular disorders. They are thought to develop from the fusion of contiguous arms of kinked segments of a capillary.

Microaneurysms may occur at any level between the superficial and deeper retinal capillary networks or even from the choroidal circulation, though the inner nuclear layer is the usual location. They vary in size from around 10 to 100 μm but only those greater than 30 μm are visible clinically. The ETDRS gives an upper limit of 125 μm diameter and the requirement of sharp borders to be considered a microaneurysm.

Larger red spots would be considered to be haemorrhages. Usually microaneurysms appear as bright red spots but occasionally they appear yellowish due to endothelial lining proliferation and hyalinization of their cavities. They may well be associated with circinate exudates.

Mild NPDR

Close examination of Fig. 7.1 reveals widely scattered microaneurysms more noticeable in the superior half of the image. Notice also the large physiologically cupped optic disc.

Mild to moderate NPDR

Intra-retinal haemorrhages appear secondary to ruptured microaneurysms, capillaries and venules. Their appearance and therefore their classification depends on their location within the retinal layers. The changes as seen in Fig. 7.2 are consistent with mild NPDR but depending on the presence of other haemorrhages elsewhere this could be classified as moderate NPDR as in Fig. 7.3.

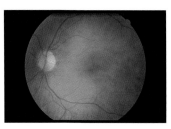

Fig. 7.1   Very mild NPDR — microaneurysms.

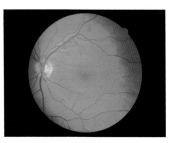

Fig. 7.2   Mild to moderate NPDR.

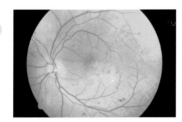

Fig. 7.3 Moderate NPDR — note dot and blot haemorrhages.

Flame-shaped haemorrhages (FSHs) occur in the superficial nerve fibre layer where the blood tends to follow the course of the nerve fibres. A FSH can be seen approximately 1 DD from the disc at 1 o'clock in Fig. 7.2.

Dot haemorrhages (Figs. 7.2 and 7.3) are located in the outer-plexiform and inner nuclear layers of the retina. Two-dot haemorrhages can be seen at approximately 5 o'clock and about 1.5 DD from the disc. On fluorescein angiography dot haemorrhages exhibit hypofluorescence as opposed to hyperfluorescence of microaneurysms. Dot haemorrhages can be indistinguishable from microaneurysms on fundoscopy.

Blot haemorrhages (as seen at the top of Fig. 7.2 and inferiorly in Fig. 7.3) are similar to dot haemorrhages but with less distinct borders. These originate from the deep capillary plexus. They are located in the inner plexiform and outer plexiform layers of the retina. Due to the compact structure of the retinal elements in this region and the relative depth at these locations, the haemorrhages assume a dark, blot-like appearance (Figs. 7.4 and 7.5). They are easily differentiated from the brighter red, flame-shaped retinal haemorrhages.

Some haemorrhages have white centres due to the presence of platelets and fibrin. Intra-retinal haemorrhages are usually found scattered throughout the posterior pole and usually resolve within 4–6 months. Haemorrhages can of course be caused by many other conditions.

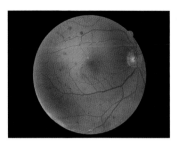

Fig. 7.4 Dot and blot haemorrhages.

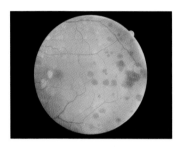

Fig. 7.5 Blot haemorrhages.

Moderate NPDR

Hard exudates (which may also be seen in mild NPDR) consist of accumulated and condensed plasma and so are made up of mainly serum lipoproteins. They represent a leakage from the circulation at a level which probably requires a degree of structural damage to vascular endothelium. Capillaries with microaneurysms are the principal source.

As exudates become progressively concentrated they give rise to semi-solid residues that acquire a characteristic hard or waxy appearance (Fig. 7.6). Hard exudates as seen in the top left of Fig. 7.6 consist of accumulated and condensed plasma and so are made up of mainly serum lipoproteins.

Fluid plasma leaks through the abnormal permeable vascular wall and seeps into the outer-plexiform layer where it collects. It is thought that the inter-photoreceptor Muller cell junctional complexes present an obstacle to the further movement of molecules the size of lipids and proteins, whilst allowing the unimpeded passage of water towards the choroid. The exudate becomes progressively concentrated to leave semi-solid residues which acquire a characteristic hard or waxy appearance.

Hard exudates may be re-absorbed either spontaneously or following laser photocoagulation. This is due to phagocytosis by macrophages. The circinate exudates in Fig. 7.6 are predominantly in the upper nasal quadrant and well away from the macula. There are a few small discrete circinate exudates within the superior temporal arcade but these are just outside a disc diameter from the fovea and so do not yet constitute a referable maculopathy. However this would require careful monitoring and the patient should be examined within 6 months.

Cotton wool spots (Fig. 7.7). These are a common feature in DR and are a consequence of capillary occlusion in the nerve fibre layer and are arranged along its long axis. This results in a stasis of axoplasmic flow within nerve fibres and a subsequent swelling of the neural tissue supplied by the arteriole. This gives rise to the fluffy white cotton wool-like lesions seen on

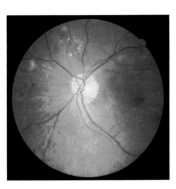

Fig. 7.6 Moderate NPDR with hard exudates.

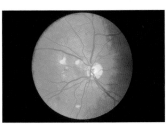

Fig. 7.7 Cotton wool spots.

fundoscopy. Most cotton wool spots have fairly common dimensions, being less than half a disc diameter in size. On very rare occasions they can be much larger ranging in size from 2 to 4 DDs according to one recent report in the literature. Cotton wool spots are almost always confined to the area adjacent to the major vascular arcades of the posterior pole (Fig. 7.8). Although not well illustrated here, small superficial FSHs are often related to cotton wool spots. Macroaneurysms may also sometimes be seen in hypertensive patients with DR (Fig. 7.9). These are essentially a feature of moderate to severe NPDR (pre-proliferative) as well as high blood pressure and can be an important sign of advancing or rapidly progressing retinopathy, as may occur in pregnancy or when high blood sugar levels are brought rapidly under control. At the bottom of Fig. 7.8 are two cotton wool spots with a third adjacent to the superior retinal artery bifurcation in the top right of the picture. However less than five cotton wool spots are often considered as part of a non-proliferative (background) retinopathy scenario in screening

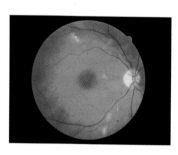

Fig. 7.8 Cotton wool spots within vascular arcades.

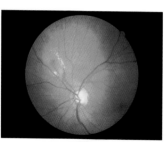

Fig. 7.9 Macroaneurysm.

protocols provided other pre-proliferative changes are not also present.

Pre-proliferative DR

The term 'pre-proliferative diabetic retinopathy' is used to describe a clinically identifiable stage of retinopathy that precedes and predicts PDR. It is characterized by significant retinal ischaemia which reflects the underlying condition of retinal capillary closure. It is important to be able to recognize this stage because patients can quickly progress to PDR.

Venous changes

Tortuosity and dilatation occur when there is sluggish retinal circulation and are the most important signs of pre-proliferative disease. Beading and looping are caused by increasing hypoxia. Focal vitreous traction may contribute to the formation of venous loops. Beading is the most important sign (Fig. 7.10).

Intra-retinal microvascular anomalies (IRMA) are a hallmark of severe NPDR and they are a precursor to PDR. Today IRMA and intra-retinal new vessels are considered to be the same. By definition, intra-retinal new vessels are IRMA as long as they are not breaking through the internal limiting membrane. In Fig. 7.11 there is an area of IRMA extending throughout the upper left quadrant indicated by the arrow. Progressive vessel damage leads to blood being forced along alternative routes i.e. via capillary networks not intended for such increased blood flows. This can result in capillary distension and irregularity.

Blot haemorrhages are another important feature seen in pre-proliferative retinopathy as seen in Fig. 7.8 adjacent to the area of IRMA and scattered throughout all four quadrants in Fig. 7.12. Note also the two cotton wool spots superiorly in Fig. 7.12.

Beading is clearly demonstrated along the vein seen in Fig. 7.10 as well as looping marked by the arrow.

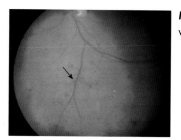

Fig. 7.10 Pre-proliferative DR with venous beading.

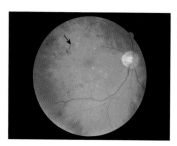

Fig. 7.11 Pre-proliferative retinopathy. (Note IRMA superiorly.)

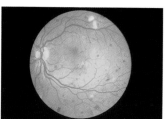

Fig. 7.12 Pre-proliferative DR. (Note multiple dot and blot haemorrhages in all four quadrants and the cotton wool spots.)

Diabetic maculopathy (DM)

DR is well recognized as the commonest cause of blindness in the working age group (20–65 years) in the United Kingdom. It is responsible for 12% of all new cases of blindness in America each year. One of the ways in which blindness occurs is when the central macular area of the retina is damaged, causing diabetic maculopathy (DM). Increased permeability of retinal vessels allows leakage of plasma constituents which accumulate in the extracellular spaces, initially at the outer-plexiform layer and inner nuclear layer level and later extending to involve the entire retinal thickness. Such oedema at the macula is the most common cause of reduced vision in NPDR.

The frequency of maculopathy varies between type 1 and type 2 diabetes and their duration. DM is more common in type 2 diabetes compared with type 1. In both types however the cumulative risk rises to approximately 30% after 20 years' duration. Other risk factors include pregnancy, hypertension, poor glycaemic control, renal disease and hyperlipidaemia.

The underlying changes which occur in DM are the same as in NPDR, although they are classified separately due to the special anatomy and function of the macula. The macula is defined as the central area of retina between the superior and inferior temporal arcades, from the disc and 2-DDs temporal to the fovea.

Oedema is difficult to see using direct ophthalmoscopy without binocular cues. Using an aspheric (e.g. Volk) lens (e.g. 78D or 90D) with slit-lamp biomicroscopy makes this easier to appreciate, although the best stereoscopic view is achieved using a fundus contact lens.

Classification of DM

There are four main types of maculopathy according to clinical examination and fluorescein angiography. These are:

- **Focal:** Leakage from dilated segments of capillaries and microaneurysms.
- **Diffuse:** Characterized by the presence of diffuse oedema.
- **Ischaemic:** Capillary shut down results in retinal non-perfusion and ischaemia. It is chararacterized by the presence of large blot haemorrhages, multiple cotton wool spots and IRMAs.
- **Mixed:** It is not uncommon to see a combination of focal, diffuse and ischaemic maculopathy.

Clinically significant macular oedema vs. referable maculopathy

Diabetic macular oedema according to the ETDRS can be defined as hard exudates and retinal thickening involving the macular area. Clinically significant macular oedema (CSMO) is defined as any one of the following:

1. retinal thickening at or within 500 μm of the centre of the macula;
2. hard exudates at or within 500 μm of the centre of the macula if associated with adjacent retinal thickening;
3. a zone or zones of retinal thickening one disc area in size at least part of which is within one DD of the centre of the fovea.

In most English screening protocols referable maculopathy is defined as any exudates or haemorrhages within one DD of the fovea (Fig. 7.13). This is different to the definition of CSMO.

Early non-referable maculopathy

In mild NPDR as seen in Fig. 7.13, the earliest visible changes that develop are microaneurysms, usually in the area temporal to the fovea. At this early stage macular oedema with retinal thickening or hard exudate formation is rare but may be a threat to macular function (Fig. 7.14). It is quite common for patients to develop one or two microaneurysms or an isolated dot haemorrhage at

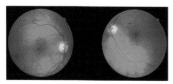

Fig. 7.13   Early maculopathy.

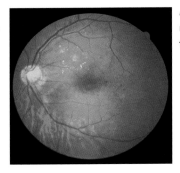

Fig. 7.14 Early non-referable maculopathy. (Note temporal fine circinate exudates.)

the macula but with no clinically significant macular oedema. Such patients do not require referral yet, but do require follow-up every 6 months. If macular oedema (thickening) becomes clinically significant then laser treatment should be undertaken.

Established focal DM

The features are well-defined focal areas of leakage with microaneurysms, haemorrhages and retinal thickening. These areas are often surrounded by circinate hard exudates. Fig. 7.15 shows a focal area of leakage with microaneurysms, haemorrhages and retinal thickening. This area is surrounded by circinate hard exudates. Note also the cluster of dot haemorrhages just temporal to the macula.

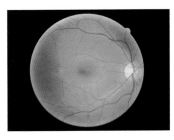

Fig. 7.15 Early referable maculopathy with circinates — just within one DD.

With focal exudative macular oedema, discrete leakage sites are a consistent feature. Leakage may occur from retinal microaneurysms or areas of dilated retinal capillaries.

The extent of the vascular changes can vary considerably. Leakage from capillaries can occur from the deep or superficial capillary network in the retina. Leakage from either microvascular abnormality gives rise to intra-retinal oedema with a bulk fluid flow towards competent capillaries. At these sites the fluid is reabsorbed into the relatively normal retinal capillary bed, causing the deposition and accumulation of the large molecules such as proteins and lipids which are seen as hard exudates.

The exact configuration of the exudate depends not only on the degree and sites of leakage, but also on the characteristics of fluid movement and absorption. Therefore exudates found at the macula vary considerably as seen in Fig. 7.16. Both these cases require referral for focal laser treatment.

In many patients with focal exudative macular oedema the areas of leakage are well away from the fovea and central vision is preserved. This is where macular oedema is not clinically significant. Most patients in this group are asymptomatic, although some may suddenly notice fluctuations in their vision or even paracentral scotoma. In patients who do suffer with disturbed central vision, the degree of visual loss is usually related to the extent of retinal oedema and hard exudate formation. Once

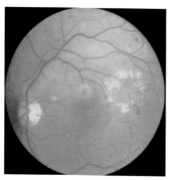

Fig. 7.16   Referable exudative DM.

retinal thickening or hard exudates are coming as close as 500 μm to the centre of the fovea, focal laser treatment is advised, even in patients with perfect vision.

Effects of statins on diabetic exudative maculopathy

When serum lipids, particularly triglycerides, increase substantially in a diabetic patient the prevalence of hard exudates increases. There is now mounting evidence that lipid-lowering drugs such as the statins can reduce the extent of macular hard exudates in patients with DR. However reducing hard exudates does not necessarily induce improved vision.

Proliferate diabetic retinopathy (PDR)

PDR is characterized by development of new vessels from the surface of the retina or optic disc as a result of retinal ischaemia. New vessels represent a serious threat to vision because they can bleed, causing pre-retinal and vitreous haemorrhages. Fibrous tissue accompanies the development of the new vessels and can lead to tractional retinal detachment.

Optic disc neovascularization (NVD) in a diabetic subject generally indicates advanced DR with retinal ischaemia and is an indication for pan-retinal photocoagulation (PRP). It is uncommon to see NVD when the area of capillary non-perfusion is less than a quarter of the whole retina.

NVD may extend over the surface of the disc and across the disc margin in one or more quadrants as seen in Fig. 7.17. Often NVD follows the retinal vessels, especially along the temporal arcades. At the advancing edge of each vessel is a loop, the tip of which serves as a focus for new growth and extension of the vessel. The fact that the advancing edges of the NVD in Fig. 7.17 are blurred is an indication that the NVDs are not all in the plane of the retina but actually also growing forwards. The vessels usually grow between the internal limiting membrane of the retina and posterior vitreous face to which they eventually become adherent. Fibrous tissue accompanies the development of the new vessels and becomes progressively more clinically obvious as seen here, superiorly to the disc.

NVD may be derived from the retinal or choroidal circulation, although it is more likely to be from the choroidal circulation if the new vessels originate from the deeper part of the cup. It is, however, difficult to be absolutely sure of the exact origin of the vessels and in any case makes no difference to the clinical management.

In the early stages it is easy to confuse NVD with fine, slightly dilated disc capillaries or even small disc collaterals. NVD does not however develop in the absence of signs of retinal ischaemia. On fluorescein angiography NVDs show leakage, whereas IRMA, collaterals and dilated disc capillaries do not.

New vessels elsewhere

New vessels elsewhere (NVE) nearly always develop from the venous sides of the capillary network adjacent to an area of retinal ischaemia. Note that the isolated NVE in Fig. 7.18 is

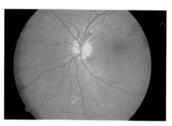

Fig. 7.17   Disc new vessels - superiorly and inferiorly.

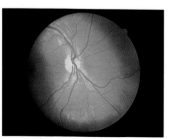

Fig. 7.18   Nasal isolated NVE.

located on the nasal fundus with very little other evidence of retinopathy present (featureless DR — see later section). This is quite a common presentation in type 1 diabetics with retinopathy. In certain camera-based diabetic screening programmes, only one fundus picture is recorded, usually including the disc, macula and temporal arcades. This case highlights the importance of always checking the nasal fundus. Had this not been the case, this relatively young patient would have been graded as mild NPDR when in fact they have proliferative disease requiring treatment.

Spontaneous regression of new vessels

There have been a few reports in the literature describing unusual spontaneous regression of new vessels. When this does occur it is often associated with improving metabolic control or at the end of a pregnancy. In other very rare cases these have been reported in type 1 diabetes in non-pregnant females with no notable improvement in their overall control of their diabetes. Such improvements are associated with a marked improvement in blood-retinal barrier breakdown and, remarkably, re-perfusion of areas of capillary dropout observed on fluorescein angiography.

Pre-retinal haemorrhage

The dark mass of blood in this characteristic (boat) shape as seen in Fig. 7.19 is a pre-retinal haemorrhage, with the blood settling in the space between the retina and vitreo-retinal membrane. The haemorrhage has a flat top due to the blood settling under the force of gravity. Although not discernible in the photograph, there must be leaking NVEs to produce this pre-retinal haemorrhage. In Fig. 7.20 extensive pre-retinal haemorrhages can be seen.

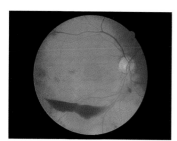

Fig. 7.19 Pre-retinal haemorrhage.

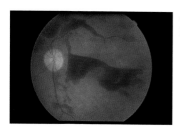

Fig. 7.20 Extensive pre-retinal haemorrhages.

Subsequent development of untreated NVD

Signs of **activity** in new vessels include neovascular buds and paucity of fibrous tissue.

Signs of **inactive** new vessels include general reduction in vascular calibre in both the new vessels and the neighbouring retinal vessels with increase in the fibrous component in the new vessels.

Potential consequences of untreated PDR

Vitreous haemorrhage occurs as a result of vitreous traction on any pre-retinal neovascular proliferation. This may result in obscuration of the fundus view in severe cases. Where the fundus cannot be visualized a B scan ultrasound can be performed to exclude any other significant pathology such as retinal detachment.

Fibrovascular tissue may shrink causing contraction and distortion of the normal retinal tissue. Combined with the process of vitreous detachment, this may progress to a tractional retinal detachment and normally affects the temporal arcades first. Temporal tractional detachments may remain more localized and do not significantly affect vision.

Tractional retinal detachments may also develop retinal tears and breaks which often result in a rapidly progressing combined tractional-rhegmatogenous retinal detachment.

Tractional retinal detachments are typically concave compared with rhegmatogenous retinal detachments that are usually convex. Also, tractional retinal detachments tend not to extend beyond the orra serrata.

Vision is significantly affected if there is foveal involvement following detachment. The vision may also be affected in other situations such as when fibrovascular tissue grows over the foveal area but with the fovea still attached. In other situations, extra-foveal fibrovascular tissue may cause tangential tractional forces giving rise to displacement of the fovea horizontally.

Rubeosis iridis is a complication of PDR in response to significant ischaemia. New vessels grow over the surface of the iris. It is therefore important to check the iris-pupil margin carefully for any signs of rubeosis in diabetics. If the new vessels obstruct the anterior chamber angles, this may lead to neovascular glaucoma.

Ocular conditions affecting DR

DR seems to show less progression in myopic eyes. Myopia of -2.00 dioptres or less is thought to be protective against development of PDR in type 1 diabetics. Proposed mechanisms of protection have included posterior vitreous detachment (PVD), decreased ocular blood flow, thinning of the retina, thereby increasing oxygen diffusion, and improved pressure dissipation by the arteriolar tree. Eyes with DR probably have shorter axial lengths than eyes without retinopathy, even in non-myopic patients with the disease.

Glaucoma and DR

Glaucoma has long been suspected to reduce the prevalence and severity of DR. This may be explained by reduced retinal metabolic activity in the retina due to decreasing viable ganglion cells and/or due to reduced vascular perfusion due to increased intraocular pressure. Similarly optic atrophy may have a protective effect against development of DR because of the reduced metabolic demand of the retina in this condition.

Posterior vitreous detachment (PVD)

The role of vitreo-retinal traction in the evolution of DR is well established. Where total PVD occurs in an eye with early NPDR, this may prevent the progression of the DR. There may well be other mechanisms present in myopic eyes.

Retinitis pigmentosa (RP) and DR

Rods have the highest metabolic rate of any cell in the body using up significant amounts of oxygen from the inner retina, rendering it almost pathologically anoxic in dark adaptation. In RP the rods degenerate and therefore reduce the demands for oxygen in the inner retina, thus reducing the risk of vasogenic cytokine release which has an important role in the pathogenesis of DR.

Atypical features of DR

'Featureless retina'

Occasionally, retinal NVD appears in patients with DR who show no other signs of intra-retinal microvascular abnormalities usually associated with pre-proliferative retinopathy (Fig. 7.21). This can be explained by the fact that cotton wool spots are transient

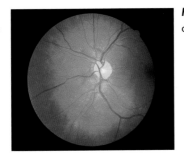

Fig. 7.21 'Featureless' DR with one isolated inferior NVE.

anyway and/or by the fact that microaneurysms, dot and blot haemorrhages and other microvascular abnormalities tend to disappear in areas of extensive capillary closure. When featureless retinae are scrutinized, they do appear to be atrophic and fluorescein angiography often reveals extensive areas of capillary non-perfusion often with previously undetected areas of NVD.

Asymmetric DR

Asymmetric DR occurs in approximately 5–10% of diabetics. It has been defined as PDR in one eye and NPDR in the other eye, persisting for more than 2 years. However it is very important not to mistake featureless retina for NPDR. There are many factors which may contribute to asymmetric DR. These include previous cataract surgery and presence of branch retinal vein occlusion.

Conversely chorioretinal scarring, optic atrophy, posterior vitreous detachment, myopia and glaucoma tend to reduce the disease progression.

Carotid occlusive disease

Where patients present with severe carotid artery stenosis, this can also be associated with worsening of the DR on the occluded side. It is thought that the carotid stenosis in effect has a

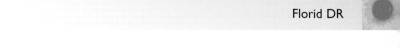

macroangiopathy which exacerbates the DR microangiopathy. When severe enough to result in ocular ischaemic syndrome, this may be indistinguishable from PDR. It is important to recognize ocular ischaemic syndrome in DR because of the poor visual prognosis if rubeosis becomes established. Where there is only mild carotid insufficiency the effect of progression on DR is less clear.

Peripheral abnormalities in DR

In a small number of cases there is a relative sparing of the posterior pole and new vessels may develop only in the far periphery where they can be easily missed. NVD of the disc may also occur even when macular and peripheral retina are well perfused. Neovascular glaucoma and anterior hyaloid fibrovascular proliferation are most likely caused by peripheral retinal ischaemia. Peripheral new vessels have certainly been reported growing from the choroid in an eye enucleated for PDR with neovascular glaucoma.

Florid DR

Florid DR (Fig. 7.22) is a rare complication of severe diabetes mellitus typically occurring in type 1 diabetics with long-standing

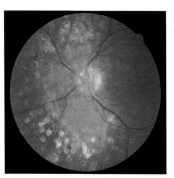

Fig. 7.22 Extensive florid NVDs post PRP.

poor control, affecting women more than men. Other systemic complications are common. This condition is encountered in less than 1% of cases with PDR. Florid DR is characterized by bilateral, rapidly progressive, severe ischaemic retinopathy associated with loss of vision and a very high risk of subsequent blindness. Therefore early detection is crucial; PRP is required with early vitrectomy when indicated to improve prognosis.

Diabetic retinal pigment epitheliopathy

Although diabetic macular oedema is mainly thought to be associated with a vascular origin, the retinal pigment epithelium may also play an important role. A disruption of the outer blood-retinal barrier may contribute to the development of DM. This is through diffuse late-phase leakage from the macular retinal pigment epithelium

Cilio-retinal artery and DM

It is often stated that the presence of a cilio-retinal artery has certain advantages regarding vascular perfusion. However where DR is concerned there may be distinct disadvantages, particularly where asymmetric retinopathy is present. This is where these vessels may be the cause of an increased prevalence of dot and blot haemorrhages, hard exudates and maculopathy with CSMO in certain patients.

Conclusion

It was the initial observation that eyes with extensive chorioretinal scarring from any cause were much less likely to develop DR, or if they did for it to be less severe, which led to the iatrogenic induction of chorioretinal scarring that paved the way for the development of PRP treatment.

The identification and better understanding of some of the less common features of DR may similarly open new as yet undiscovered treatment options for such retinal disease.

Further reading

Akduman L, Olk R J 1995 The early treatment of diabetic retinopathy study. In: Kertes P J, Conway M D (eds) 1998 *Clinical trials in ophthalmology – a summary and practice guide*, Chapter 2. Pennsylvania, USA: Lippincott Williams & Wilkins

Benson W 2000 Diabetic retinopathy. In: Yanoff M, Duker J S (eds) *Ophthalmology*. New York, USA: Mosby

Hamilton A M P, Ulbig M W, Polkinghorne P 1996 Management of diabetic retinopathy. In: Hamilton (ed) *Lesions of diabetic retinopathy*. London: BMJ Publishing Group, p 96–156

Harvey W 1997 Background diabetic retinopathy (parts 1&2). *Diabetes module parts 1–12 continuing professional development series*. London: Association of Optometrists and City University

Kanski J 2003 *Clinical ophthalmology: a systematic approach*, 5th edn. London: Butterworth Heinemann

8
Management of diabetic retinopathy and diabetic maculopathy — laser, surgical and medical approaches

Introduction

A number of large randomized controlled trials have demonstrated the benefit of treating patients with diabetic retinopathy (DR) using retinal photocoagulation with laser and vitrectomy surgery. This chapter describes the indications, techniques and results of treatment with these modalities. However it should also be remembered that, to effectively manage DR, it is also important to:

- optimize glucose control;
- detect sight-threatening retinopathy promptly by means of an effective screening system and to provide careful follow-up where appropriate;
- manage the common systemic conditions associated with diabetes including: hypertension, dyslipidaemia, anaemia and obstructive sleep apnoea (see Chapter 10);
- manage the effects of diabetes on other organs, in particular renal impairment. Diabetic nephropathy is strongly associated with sight-threatening DR and proteinuria should be screened for. Anaemia associated with nephropathy should be managed as above (see Chapter 10). Dialysis once required can often lead to a striking improvement in retinopathy, in particular where there is macular oedema;
- control other risk factors such as smoking (see Chapter 10).

Retinal photocoagulation for DR

General principles of photocoagulation

Photocoagulation is accomplished by directing a focused laser (**L**ight **A**mplification by the **S**timulated **E**mission of **R**adiation) beam of a discrete wavelength onto specified parts of the retina. Absorption in a variety of intraocular retinal layers, in particular the retinal pigment epithelium (RPE), causes a local rise in temperature of around 30°C, which in turn causes denaturation of tissue proteins and coagulative necrosis. The target and level of photocoagulation within the retina is determined by the wavelength used and pigment distribution involved. Absorbing pigments in the eye include:

- melanin in the RPE;
- xanthophyll (in the yellow macular pigment visible clinically and present in the crystalline lens);
- haemoglobin within red blood cells;
- melanin in choroidal and scleral melanocytes;
- lipofuscin in ageing eyes.

Through the use of different wavelengths of light that are selectively absorbed by RPE, retinal blood vessels or melanin, tissue effects can be induced at different levels within the retina.

Mechanisms of photocoagulation inhibiting exudation and resulting in the involution of retinal neovascularization are complex and still not completely understood, but include:

1. Laser may cause RPE-mediated release of growth factors and cytokines to restore the inner and outer blood-retinal barriers (this is commonly thought to be the most likely mode of action in diabetic maculopathy treatment).
2. Laser-induced damage to the RPE might allow movement of anti-angiogenic factors into the inner retina.
3. Improved oxygenation of the inner retina as a result of laser-induced destruction of the metabolically active RPE/photoreceptor complex. This is thought to be the likely mode of action in pan-retinal photocoagulation (PRP).

Deciding which wavelength and laser to use is an important consideration (although most units do not have a choice!).

Argon laser

Argon laser is a common laser used for treating DR. The main spectral peaks of the argon laser are 488 nm (blue) and 514 nm (green) i.e. relatively shorter wavelengths. Modern argon lasers remove blue wavelength light, allowing photocoagulation to be achieved at 514 nm which reduces light scatter as well as preventing absorption of the blue 488-nm wavelength by xanthophyll in the macula. Argon laser 514 nm without the blue 488-nm wavelength is well suited for treating diabetic maculopathy (Fig. 8.1).

Frequency-doubled YAG (532 nm) is a green wavelength similar to argon (514 nm). Many units now use this laser which, being a solid state laser system, is produced without the need for large gas laser tubes.

Diode laser

Diode laser (810 nm) has less uptake by haemoglobin, allowing laser through light vitreous haemorrhages, whilst maintaining a fairly high uptake in melanin. One disadvantage is that it tends to produce deeper burns with potentially more pain and a harder visible end point to define clinically whilst undertaking the laser treatment, i.e. greyer, less white, burns.

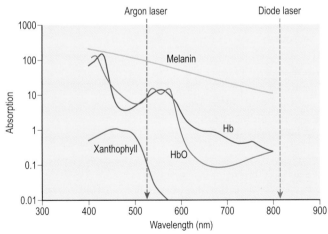

Fig. 8.1 Absorption characteristics of argon and diode lasers.

A relatively selective RPE effect can be produced by using a micro-pulse mode delivering the laser energy in very narrow pulses that can still produce a retinal pigment epithelial burn whilst greatly reducing the surrounding spread of energy to adjacent tissues (see later in new treatments section).

Instrumentation

Lasers are usually attached to a modified slit-lamp biomicroscope (Fig. 8.2) and the laser light is directed into the eye through a diagnostic contact lens (e.g. an Area Centralis or Quadraspheric lens — Fig. 8.3). Many modern lasers have a coaxial red wavelength

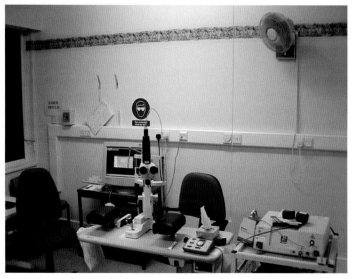

Fig. 8.2 Laser room set up — note solid state double frequency YAG laser, monitor to show fundal images and cooling fan!

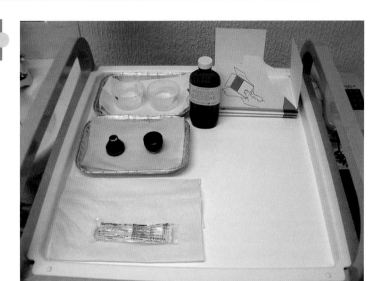

Fig. 8.3 Diagnostic laser lenses — note lenses are cleaned as per a prescribed protocol in between patients.

laser as an aiming beam. Also there are filters incorporated into the optical system, which prevent reflected laser light and flashbacks which could potentially cause damage to the operator's eye. Portable systems are also now available which run off standard mains electricity supply, making laser treatment during peripheral outreach clinics and non-hospital environments possible.

Indications for laser treatment in DR

Indications for laser treatment of DR include photocoagulation for:

- diabetic maculopathy;
- proliferative retinopathy.

Diabetic maculopathy

Aims of laser treatment in diabetic maculopathy

Diabetic maculopathy, i.e. diabetic retinopathy affecting the macular area of the retina, is the commonest cause of reduced vision in patients with diabetic retinopathy. Laser treatment of diabetic maculopathy has been shown to be effective in preventing visual loss in several large clinical randomized trials, however it is not a cure and cannot prevent loss of vision in all patients.

Retinal microvascular damage results in reduced function in the parts of the retina affected. Hence severe microvascular damage at the foveal centre will result in significantly impaired vision whilst less severe and more eccentric microvascular changes may be completely asymptomatic. The extent of microvascular damage can range from mild capillary wall incompetence with leakage to complete capillary occlusion. Clinically, maculopathy can therefore be categorized by the exact area of macula affected and divided up into three types by the degree of vascular damage:

1. **exudative** which can be either focal or diffuse with or without exudates;
2. **ischaemic** with capillary closure;
3. **mixed**.

Laser treatment for diabetic maculopathy aims to arrest leakage from microvascular abnormalities (mainly microaneurysms and areas of diffuse capillary wall leakage) to allow fluid and hard exudates to re-absorb. It cannot be applied to the foveal centre and cannot improve ischaemia. Hence the efficacy of laser treatment is dependent on the type and location of maculopathy and the extent of visual loss already present. Essentially patients with eccentric disease and microvascular leak, where the foveal centre is unaffected, are at risk from becoming oedematous from the eccentric leaking areas. These patients stand most to gain from focal laser treatment.

Treatment is therefore given in patients with some degree of exudative maculopathy primarily to reduce the risk of visual loss occurring by macular oedema involving the foveal centre.

The risk of moderate visual loss (doubling of the visual angle) can be very approximately quantified into three depending on the type of maculopathy present:

1. focally exudative maculopathy with circinate exudates: the prognosis is best with only approximately 10% of patients suffering moderate visual loss within 1 year;
2. diffusely oedematous maculopathy: prognosis is worse with 20% experiencing moderate visual loss in 1 year;
3. ischaemic maculopathy: 30% will suffer moderate visual loss within 1 year.

Year on year there is a gradual increase in the risk of moderate visual loss and the control arm of the Early Treatment Diabetic Retinopathy Study (ETDRS) gives useful natural history data on the risk of visual loss in the first 3 years once macular oedema develops (Table 8.1) The ETDRS natural history data can be further broken down to look at the figures for those patients in which foveal involvement was present from the onset (Table 8.2). These show that the risks of moderate visual loss were significantly increased if this was present. Of course patients with diabetic maculopathy can also get a gradual deterioration in their level of retinopathy. If clinically significant macular oedema is present, then approximately 25% of patients will go on to get

Table 8.1   ETDRS results for laser for maculopathy

	1 year	2 year	3 year
With laser	5%	7%	12%
Without (natural history)	8%	16%	24%

Note: 1) Results are given as percentage of patients experiencing moderate visual loss; 2) improvement in 'appearance' in 65–100% of cases; 3) 35% of eyes in ETDRS were non-CSMO.

Table 8.2 ETDRS results for laser for maculopathy with foveal involvement

	1 year	2 year
With laser	13%	20%
Without (natural history)	33%	54%

Results are given as percentage of patients experiencing moderate visual loss.

high-risk proliferative diabetic retinopathy within 5 years. In patients with diffuse maculopathy and foveal involvement this figure is approximately 40–50%.

Retinal thickening and exudation can be identified by clinical examination. The decision whether to start treatment (looking at the degree and location of retinal thickening and exudation) is based on the findings of the ETDRS which defined so-called "clinically significant macular oedema" (i.e. maculopathy where vision is likely to deteriorate in the near future) as exudates **associated with** thickening or thickening on its own within 500 microns from the foveal centre, or an area of thickening at least **one disc area in size** within 1500 microns from the foveal centre, i.e.:

1. thickening of the retina located < or = to 500 microns from the centre of the fovea;
2. hard exudates with thickening of the adjacent retina located < or = 500 microns from the centre of the fovea;
3. a zone or retinal thickening, one disc area or larger in size located < or = one disc diameter (~1500 microns) from the centre of the fovea.

Note that it is the clinical appearance and not the fluorescein angiography appearance that is the cue to commence treatment.

In the ETDRS, treatment with immediate focal or grid-pattern laser photocoagulation significantly reduced the incidence of moderate visual loss compared to the sub-group in which focal laser photocoagulation for macular oedema was deferred. Immediate photocoagulation reduced the incidence of moderate visual loss by ~50% at all time points, compared with treatment deferral. After 3 years follow up, 12% of eyes with CSMO had moderate visual loss as opposed to 24% in the untreated control group.

When to treat focal maculopathy
Patients with macular oedema or hard exudates not in the foveal area, or encroaching on the fovea, can usually be carefully followed up without undertaking laser treatment. Once there is definite evidence of progression with CSMO, laser treatment should be undertaken.

In practice thresholds for treatment may be lowered in a number of other situations including:

1. if PRP is planned (as this can exacerbate macular oedema);
2. if cataract surgery is being planned (as this can also potentially exacerbate macular oedema);
3. if early worsening of retinopathy is anticipated following a tightening of glucose control;
4. if the patient becomes pregnant, as retinopathy can progress significantly during pregnancy;
5. if a patient has a history of poor attendance.

Fluorescein angiography
Intravenous fluorescein angiography (IVFA) is not undertaken in all cases, although as part of good clinical practice colour photographs should always be taken before treatment. IVFA is useful in cases where:

- the area of leakage is uncertain;
- the exact location of the leaking areas with respect to the foveal centre is uncertain;
- there is diffuse macular oedema with foveal centre involvement;
- the extent of capillary closure is uncertain but clinically suspected when there are multiple retinal haemorrhages, surprisingly reduced visual acuity, cotton wool spots and little if any exudates (Fig. 8.4);
- other pathology is suspected; and in
- non-responsive cases and re-treatments.

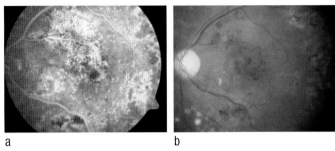

a   b

Fig. 8.4   Mixed ischaemic and exudative maculopathy — note confluent blotch haemorrhages in ischaemic area with possible additional branch retinal vein occlusion.

Microaneurysms show up as tiny 'balloons' in the early phases of an angiogram. Microaneurysms that are leaking can be identified in the later stages with leaking fluorescein spreading centrifugally. Fluorescein angiography also may help locate the foveal avascular zone (FAZ), which may be difficult to accurately locate clinically because of overlying macular oedema. Areas of capillary dropout that have macular oedema can be identified as dark areas of avascular retina (Fig. 8.5). Dilated capillaries that leak show up as diffuse areas of fluorescence in the later stages of the angiogram, with vessel wall staining.

Patterns of laser treatment for maculopathy
The choice of treatment application is dependent on the extent and pattern of macula oedema and the extent of the lesions being treated. Laser treatment is effective for oedematous maculopathies either focal or diffuse, with or without exudates.

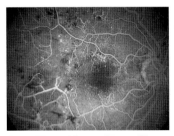

Fig. 8.5   Angiogram demonstrating temporal ischaemia with multiple microvascular abnormalities, venous beading and venous loop formation.

It is also effective in mixed maculopathies with ischaemic and exudative components, but is not effective in purely ischaemic maculopathies.

Laser treatment for maculopathy is generally applied to areas of vascular leakage in one of the following patterns:

- **Focal** — This is used for circumscribed small areas of macular oedema where laser burns are applied to areas of micro-aneurysms and microvascular lesions in the centre of rings of hard exudates (Fig. 8.6). Burns are commonly 100 microns in diameter with 0.08–0.1 second duration. Longer burn duration causes bigger burns and increased inner retinal damage by thermal spread and shorter burns risk causing intense effects with bruchs membrane fractures, risk of haemorrhage and later choroidal neovascularization. The power is measured in milliwatts and should be kept as low as possible, typically starting at around 100 mW. Light burns are therefore used so that the laser reaction is just visible as a faint greyish-white reaction — a threshold burn. Generally no attempt is made to close retinal blood vessels. A suitable contact viewing lens is selected and placed on the eye with hydroxymethylcellulose or other suitable gel as a coupling agent.

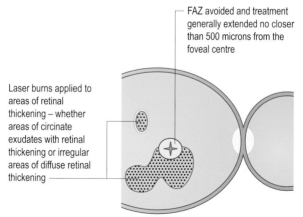

FAZ avoided and treatment generally extended no closer than 500 microns from the foveal centre

Laser burns applied to areas of retinal thickening – whether areas of circinate exudates with retinal thickening or irregular areas of diffuse retinal thickening

Fig. 8.6 Diagrammatic representation of focal/modified grid laser.

- **Grid** — This is used when there is generalized diffuse macular oedema with foveolar involvement (Fig. 8.6), typically using a spot size of 100–200 microns with a grid pattern of 100–200 burns of 0.08–1.0 s duration around the macula. The burns should be of light intensity and placed approximately one burn-width apart. If treatment is taken into areas with less macular oedema, then the power setting should be reduced. Treatment closer than 500 microns from the FAZ should be undertaken with caution but is occasionally done as repeat treatment in non-responsive cases with persistent central oedema. The papillomacular bundle area can be safely treated provided there is macular oedema within this area, as in this situation the nerve fibre layer will be separated from the area of maximum energy uptake within the RPE and thus protected from thermal damage. Care should therefore be taken in treating 'dry' retina within this area and in re-treatments.
- **Modified grid** is similar to grid settings except the pattern is concentrated in a particular sector or sectors of retinal thickening rather than a general pattern around the foveal centre (Figs. 8.6 and 8.7). In practice this pattern of treatment rather than grid laser is more commonly applied.
- Treatment was also given in the EDTRS to areas of ecentric capillary non-perfusion associated with retinal thickening in the macular area.

Titration of laser power
Power should be titrated upwards carefully aiming for a 'just visible' burn with a slight grey appearance. Test burns can be applied on a part of the retina by the arcades and power titrated up to a grey burn, and then the thickened area treated using this power initially. Usually slightly more power will be needed in the thickened area of the retina to get the same burn intensity, but this is a safe protocol for initial power estimation. Pseudophakic eyes usually need much less power than phakic eyes because of natural lens pigment and light scatter. Treatment through a cataract is often possible but burn intensity can vary significantly as the laser passes through different parts of the cataract.

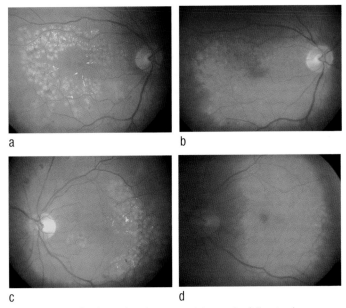

a b

c d

Fig. 8.7 (a,b,c,d) Immediately post and 6 months following laser for multifocal exudative maculopathy. Visual acuity (VA) at last follow-up 6/6 R+L.

Lower powers will be needed in highly pigmented individuals. In myopic and very lightly pigmented patients however operators should be wary of using too much power. The burns will be very difficult to see because of the lightly pigmented fundus, but paradoxically, several months after the laser reaction can be marked with large depigmented scars. These scars can also enlarge with time and can encroach upon central vision if central.

Focal laser is not usually painful; if it is then too much power is being used other than in very rare individuals.

Identifying fixation during laser treatment
At the start of each treatment session the foveal centre should be accurately identified. This can often be clinically obvious, but patients can eccentrically fixate, and it is worth identifying the fixation point as well. This can be done either by using a small

round illumination light or the aiming beam of the laser, which is red. After identifying fixation the patient should be told to look at the white fixation light with their non-treatment eye. The patient should be very clearly told at this point that the aiming beam for the laser is red and under no circumstances should they ever look at the red beam again during the treatment, as this would put them at risk of getting a foveal burn!

Patients who are extremely photophobic
Diabetic patients with retinopathy occasionally suffer from painful light sensitivity. Treatment should start with the lowest illumination levels possible and should be gradually increased to the desired level for clearly visible treatment. Sometimes patients are less photophobic with the red-free light and this can occasionally be worthwhile trying. Time must be allowed for the patient to adjust to the light. In very photophobic patients who blink each time the laser is fired, care should be taken of treating too close to the fovea, especially inferior to the fovea, because of Bell's phenomenon.

In extremely photophobic patients it is sometimes necessary to give a sub-Tenon's block, especially if treatment near the centre is required.

Three to four weeks following argon laser the laser burns can be seen as small pigmented areas on the RPE (Fig. 8.7). Patients vary greatly in the amount of reaction they develop to laser burns, ranging from barely visible reactions to quite extensive atrophic lesions. Although this is partly related to laser energy, it appears to be a fairly individual response and the appearance of the macula cannot be used to determine how strong the laser was!

Results of laser treatment for diabetic maculopathy
Usually patients should be evaluated 2–4 months after treatment. Any residual oedema should be assessed and any additional leaking points should be considered for more treatment. It is not uncommon for more retinal micro-aneurysms to be seen at this visit, because their visibility increases as the surrounding semi-opaque oedema subsides. Similarly exudates can increase temporarily and re-treatment should not be reconsidered prematurely.

The best results with focal laser are obtained in those eyes with well-defined circinate, hard exudates, of recent duration, but negligible or no involvement of the fovea and good vision. The poorest response is seen in the following eyes:

- where central vision is reduced as a result of a foveal plaque of exudates;
- where there is diffuse oedema with multiple leaking areas;
- extensive central capillary non-perfusion (Fig. 8.8);
- uncontrolled hypertension;
- long-standing cystoid macular oedema.

Unresponsive diabetic maculopathy
In patients who are unresponsive to laser, fluorescein angiography should be performed to target repeat treatment and assess the degree of ischaemia present (Fig. 8.8). There are a number of other possible causes for unresponsive maculopathies, including:

- renal impairment (dialysis can often) lead to a marked improvement in macular oedema in patients with progressive renal impairment;
- hypertension — this is often a significant problem and must be treated;
- poor diabetic control;
- vitreous traction — if this is suspected then optical coherence tomography (OCT) is very useful and the patient should be considered for vitrectomy;

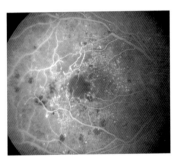

Fig. 8.8 Ischaemic maculopathy on IVFA.

- choroidal neovascularization (this should show up on angiography);
- ivenous obstruction (again this should hopefully be clarified on angiography).

Complications

Para central scotomata are common after treatment close to the foveal centre. Patients should be warned that they may notice grey scotomata around their central vision for a few days to weeks after treatment. These usually however fade with time, but not always.

Transient worsening of vision can occur due to a transient increase in oedema following treatment; again this usually improves.

Choroidal neovascularization can occur and patients should be specifically warned of this complication if they have existing age-related macular degeneration (AMD). In this situation the choroidal neovascular membrane (CNVM) can actually be just part of the AMD natural history and not part of the laser treatment (Fig. 8.9). High intensity small burns should be avoided which can rupture bruchs membrane increasing the likelihood of choroidal neovascularization. Also it should be noted that CNVM can occur spontaneously in patients with severe diabetic macular oedema (DMO).

Sub retinal fibrosis can occur, but again this can occur in diffusely oedematous maculae as part of the diabetic maculopathy disease course. Similarly **epiretinal membrane** formation can occur (Fig. 8.10).

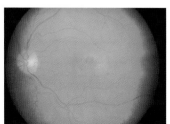

Fig. 8.9 Small choroidal neovascular membrane post focal laser treatment — there was later spontaneous regression of membrane and a return to 6/6 vision.

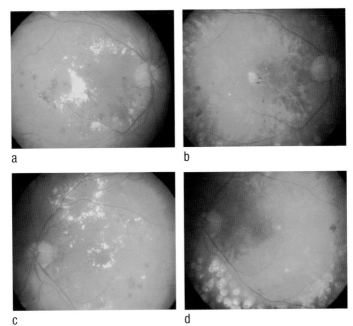

a   b

c   d

Fig. 8.10 (a,b,c,d)   Pre (upper) and post (lower) laser views of patients with PDR and severe maculopathy — note right subretinal fibrosis at site of central plaque exudate post laser.
Vas at last follow-up R 6/60, L 6/36.

Laser scar expansion can occur, especially in myopic patients as discussed above.

Exudate deposition at the foveal centre can occur in extremely oedematous retinae after treatment, and large exudates close to the fovea are also a risk factor. In patients with grossly oedematous maculae, or exudates very close to fixation, the option of fractionating the maculopathy treatment in a couple of sessions should be considered to try and avoid the risk of sub-foveal exudate deposition.

Increased ischaemia can occur rarely after maculopathy treatment, especially in patients with mixed maculopathy.

If ischaemia is suspected an angiogram should be arranged so that this complication can be discussed with the patient if they wish. This is best undertaken with the patient looking at the angiogram with the operating clinician.

Colour vision and contrast sensitivity can be reduced following laser and again should be discussed if this is relevant to the patient's profession or hobbies in particular.

Focal laser treatment for diabetic maculopathy clearly works and the commonest cause for reduction in vision following laser treatment is actually progression in maculopathy rather than deterioration in vision secondary to laser. The incidence of iatrogenic visual acuity reduction following laser is probably less than 1 in 300 in the author's (D. Steel) experience.

Laser treatment of proliferative diabetic retinopathy (PDR)

Aims of treatment

The aim of PRP laser therapy in PDR is to induce involution of new vessels thereby preventing visual loss from vitreous haemorrhage and tractional retinal detachment.

Indications for PRP

PRP significantly reduces the likelihood that an eye with retinal neovascularization will experience severe visual loss. The Diabetic Retinopathy Study (DRS) Research Group, which was one of the first randomized control trials ever undertaken in ophthalmology, conclusively demonstrated the efficacy of laser PRP in PDR. After 2 years, eyes which had received 1200–1600, 500 micron PRP burns had less than half the rate of severe vision loss compared with the control eyes that had received no laser treatment (Table 8.3). The absolute risk reduction obviously depends upon the severity and natural history risk of a particular eye with retinopathy at baseline and the DRS provided useful natural history figures for this (Table 8.4).

Both the DRS and ETDRS showed that PRP should be given promptly if certain 'high risk' features were present and this has led to a definition of 'high risk' PDR (Box 8.1).

Table 8.3   Risk of severe visual loss (VA<1/40) at 2 years

Severe NPDR	3%
NVE only	6.8%
Small NVD	10.5%
Small NVD with vitreous haemorrhage	25.6%
Severe NVD with VH	36.9%

Table 8.4   Risk of severe visual loss in PDR

Vit haem	NVs	NVD	Large NVs	No. of risk factors	2-year risk of severe visual loss
+				1	4.2
	+			1	6.8
+	+			2	6.4
	+		+	2	6.8
+	+		+	3	29.7
	+	+		2	10.5
+	+	+		3	25.6
	+	+	+	3	26.2
+	+	+	+	4	36.9

> **Box 8.1   Definition of 'high risk' proliferative retinopathy**
> The presence of any three of the following:
> - Vitreous haemorrhage.
> - New vessels.
> - NVD.
> - NVD > 1/3 DA or NVE > 1/2 DA.
>
> NVD are the single most important prognostic factor for the risk of severe visual loss in DR.

'High risk' PDR

An eye is classified as having high risk PDR if it contains any three of the following features, namely:

1. vitreous haemorrhage;
2. any new vessels;
3. new vessels at the optic disc;
4. new vessels at the optic disc greater than one-third of a disc area in size, or new vessels elsewhere greater than half a disc area in size.

The following clinical scenarios are defined as 'high risk' PDR:

1. Mild disc new vessels (NVD) less than one-third of the disc area with haemorrhage. This carries a 26% risk of severe visual loss over 2 years. This can be reduced to 4% with PRP laser treatment.
2. Severe NVD greater than half the disc area without haemorrhage. This carries a 26% risk of visual loss which is reduced to 9% with treatment.
3. Severe NVD with haemorrhage carries a 37% risk of visual loss, which reduces to 20% with treatment.
4. Severe new vessels elsewhere (NVE) greater than half a disc area with vitreous or pre-retinal haemorrhage. This carries a 30% risk of visual loss, which is reduced to 7% with treatment.

New vessels on the optic disc are thus the single most important prognostic factor for the visual prognosis in PDR.

For lesser degrees of PDR the beneficial effect of the PRP is less obvious. However, these types of retinopathy can still progress. In patients with small new vessels at the optic disc without a vitreous haemorrhage, and therefore without 'high risk' retinopathy, the risk of progression to 'high risk' retinopathy, without treatment, is 59% within 2 years versus 22% with PRP treatment.

Unless 'high risk' characteristics are present PRP may be withheld and the patient closely monitored at 3-monthly intervals. However in the UK many ophthalmologists often perform PRP treatment at the first sign of neovascularization especially if the following features are present.

1. patients are poor clinic attendees;
2. if the other eye has severe retinopathy;
3. if cataract surgery is planned;
4. if there are a number of other indicators in the retina suggestive that a large degree of ischaemia is present and that the retinopathy is highly likely to progress i.e. severe to very severe NPDR, e.g. widespread IRMA (Figs. 8.11 and 8.12);
5. retinopathy is deteriorating and metabolic control is poor.

The 1-year risk of severe NPDR progressing to high risk PDR is 15% without treatment and about 8% with PRP (Table 8.5). The beneficial effect of PRP in patients with severe NPDR is thus less

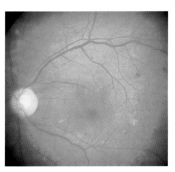

Fig. 8.11 Multiple IRMA.

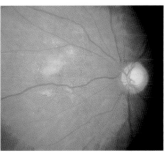

Fig. 8.12 IRMA nasally.

Table 8.5   Risk of progression to high-risk characteristics in 1 year

(All values in %)	Treated	Untreated
Severe NPDR	8.8	15
Mild NVE	8.5	19.4
Severe NVE	12.2	24.5
Mild NVD	21.9	58.7

clear and usually PRP laser treatment is not given. There are however exceptions to the rule and PRP laser treatment may be considered, as with low risk PDR, if the above features are present.

Treatment technique for PRP
A standard initial PRP is approximately 1200–1600 burns of 500 microns size (Fig. 8.13). The author (D. Steel) routinely uses a quadraspheric lens which magnifies the spot by about 2x (Table 8.6). Therefore to get a 500-micron retinal burn a 250-micron spot size needs to be selected on the laser console. Longer duration burns result in larger burns but with no more pain during treatment, and so PRP is often delivered with either a 0.03 or 0.08s duration as a compromise. A white grey burn is aimed for: more intense than focal (Fig. 8.14).

The amount of PRP in any one session is dictated by a number of factors including the patient's tolerance. In general, more initial PRP is attempted in higher risk situations, such as in patients with very high risk PDR or in patients who have a poor repeat attendance record. Less PRP is administered in one session if treatment fractionation is planned, for example if there are concerns regarding maculopathy exacerbation. In a patient with NVE only and some maculopathy it may actually be best to treat the macula first without any PRP or possibly just sector PRP around the NVE and then arrange two further PRP sessions of 700 burns each 3–4 weeks later, or possibly even when the

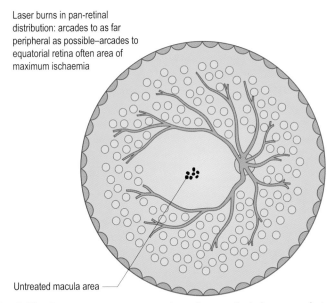

Laser burns in pan-retinal distribution: arcades to as far peripheral as possible–arcades to equatorial retina often area of maximum ischaemia

Untreated macula area

Fig. 8.13 Diagrammatic representation of pan-retinal photocoagulation (PRP).

macular is dry, if the macula is particularly oedematous. Triamcinolone given via a posterior sub-Tenon's injection before PRP can also reduce the risk of maculopathy exacerbation in this situation.

Conversely, if a patient has large new vessels at the disc with a light vitreous haemorrhage, it may be appropriate to deliver 2000 burns in one session before further haemorrhage occurs. Another strategy in this situation especially if the macula is suspect would be to give 1000 burns inferiorly and then arrange for a superior PRP 1–2 weeks later.

Similarly if a patient has iris and irido-corneal angle rubeosis, laser needs to be applied rapidly before the angle is permanently closed. Paradoxically intraocular pressure (IOP) can be raised with an open angle in an eye with angle rubeosis. These eyes often still respond well to PRP with regression of rubeotic vessels and reduced IOP. For patients with rubeosis and a hazy cornea secondary to raised IOP a useful technique is to use glycerol as

Table 8.6   Summary of lenses and treatment parameters

Lens	Magnification
Area Centralis	1 (therefore for a 100-micron burn, set laser spot size to 100 microns)
Quadraspheric	2 (therefore for a 500-micron burn, set laser spot size to 250 microns)
Super quad	2 (therefore for a 500-micron burn, set laser spot size to 250 microns)

	Burn size	Burn duration	Lens	Approx. usual power	Follow-up
Macula treatment	100–200 microns	0.08–0.1	Area Centralis	~0.07–0.2 watts	3–4 months
PRP	300–500 microns	0.03–0.08	Quadraspheric or super quad	~0.25–0.75 watts	3–6 weeks

the contact lens contact solution to keep the cornea dehydrated and clearer during treatment. The aim is to get PRP on swiftly and efficiently with a local anaesthetic block if necessary (see below).

Some patients prefer to have 500–600 burns in three to four sessions even if this means they are coming back each week for 4 weeks. Other patients may prefer to get the treatment completed in one session because of problems with transport etc.

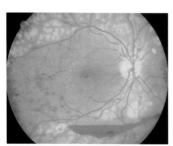

Fig. 8.14   PDR — immediately post laser.

However, if there is any degree of treatable maculopathy present it should be ensured that macular treatment is undertaken either before the PRP is started, or at the same time as the PRP. PRP can produce dramatic RPE pigmentation and hypertrophy with a 'surface of a moon' type appearance (Fig. 8.15).

Pain during PRP laser treatment
All patients get some degree of pain during a PRP, which is the main difference patients notice between focal and PRP laser! The degree of pain however is surprisingly variable between patients ranging from very mild to completely intolerable. Pain is usually greater on re-treatments, whilst treating the anterior retina, in eyes with light RPE and whilst treating the horizontal midlines where the long ciliary nerves are located.

There are a number of strategies that can be tried if pain is significant:

1. If the PRP does not need to be done quickly, fractionate the treatment in a number of divided sessions.
2. When administering the PRP it is best to leave the horizontal and peripheral retinal areas until the end.
3. Reducing the duration of the burns reduces the pain, so if a patient is experiencing pain with a 0.08-second exposure then reducing the burn duration to 0.05 seconds or even 0.03 seconds can often improve things.

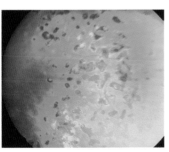

Fig. 8.15   Old PRP burns.

4. Similarly reducing spot size can sometimes reduce pain but this means that more burns need to be given to achieve the same area of retinal coverage.

5. Often pain during PRP is actually due to the contact lens being pressed hard on the eye. Additional anaesthetic drops may help and also slightly pulling the lens away from the eyeball can help, although patients that squeeze their eyelids closed during treatment will expel the lens if this is done!

6. If pain is intolerable or unpleasant then a local anaesthetic injection can be used such as a sub-Tenon's block.

7. Occasionally patients require general anaesthesia, but this is probably 1–2% of cases only. However it is better to do a PRP under a general anaesthetic (GA) than not do it at all and it is actually quite a reasonable strategy. This is especially the case in young patients with a lot of pain during laser with very high risk disease, as laser can be applied bilaterally and completely in one session.

8. Paracetamol taken before the laser session can help reduce pain and headache after the laser.

9. Inhaled entonox has also been used in some units to help pain during the laser delivery.

PRP laser distribution

Most patients with PDR have mid peripheral retinal ischaemia (essentially from the arcades to the equator). Conveniently an this is an easy area to treat (Fig. 8.15). Some patients do however have more peripheral ischaemia, especially patients with iris rubeosis and patients with gross proliferative retinopathy, and in these patients the peripheral retina should be treated as well. This can be carried out using peripheral viewing contact lenses such as a three-mirror lens or superquad. The extreme anterior retina can be treated using indirect ophthalmoscope-delivered laser and scleral indentation.

An area often undertreated is the area immediately temporal to the fovea. Treatment should be carried out to within a disc diameter of the disc nasally and PRP should be taken to within three disc diameters of the fovea temporally. With wide-angle viewing lenses such as a quadraspheric lens it is easy to keep the macula in view during this and there is less risk of foveal burns as there is when using mirrored lenses.

In patients with very severe PDR and posterior ischaemia on the angiogram (Fig. 8.16), PRP may be carried out even more posterior than this, but obviously the more posterior the PRP the more problematical peripheral field constriction can be. Very posterior fill-in should be undertaken with smaller spot sizes such as 200–300 microns.

Patients with NVE should have more treatment peripheral to the NVE than in the areas without NVE. If patients have small flat persistent peripheral NVE after full PRP with recurrent haemorrhages then the NVE can be directly treated with long duration 0.2 s and large spot size (500–600 micron burns). This strategy should be avoided with very posterior NVE because of the large scotoma produced and also avoided in NVE associated with a significant fibrous component because of the risk of exacerbating retinal traction.

Indirect ophthalmoscope-delivered laser
PRP can be delivered using an indirect ophthalmoscope system. Combined with indentation this allows more peripheral retinal treatment. It also allows treatment perioperatively, e.g. immediately after cataract extraction at the time of surgery

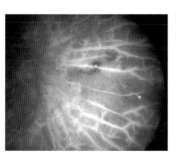

Fig. 8.16 Gross nasal retinal ischaemia on IVFA.

(Fig. 8.17). If indirect laser is performed outside of a surgical situation then the following points are useful to remember:

1. If laser uptake is impossible using a slit-lamp delivered laser because of media opacity it will not be possible using indirect laser either. Therefore consider combined cataract extraction with phacoemulsification.
2. Use local anaesthetic as laser and indentation can be painful. This can be given either as a sub-Tenon's block or, if very peripheral treatment is to be given only, then a subconjunctival injection can be a useful technique allowing the patient to gaze in the desired direction during treatment delivery.
3. The patient needs to be lying down at the correct height with good access all around their head for 360-degree treatment access.

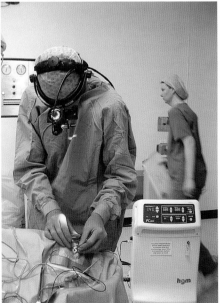

Fig. 8.17 Performing indirect argon laser with scleral indentation during surgery (note — lights on in room for photographic reasons!).

4. Use a speculum and either have an assistant to keep the cornea moistened with balanced salt solution or alternatively use hydroxymethylcellulose or hypromellose as a corneal wetting agent.

Review after PRP
Patients receiving PRP should be reviewed within 4 weeks post-treatment. Partial regression at this stage is a good sign (Fig. 8.18). Some patients may require further fill-in PRP treatment particularly if they still possess 'high-risk' PDR. Treatment may therefore be repeated and titrated according to response until up to ~6000 burns have been applied, depending on ocular size, treatment density and the diameter of the burns.

The question of whether PDR should be treated with additional fill-in treatment after an initial PRP is often, however, a difficult one. In the DRS total regression in new vessels only occurred in approximately 30–40% of all patients and partial regression occurred in a further 30–40%. A significant proportion therefore had either no reduction in size of the new vessels or an increase in size.

Elevated new vessels generally respond less well than flat new vessels. Patients can continue to get vitreous haemorrhages, despite PRP, secondary to vitreous traction. In this situation an attempt should be made to gauge whether the new vessels are actively proliferating and growing or whether it is simply vitreous traction with inactive new vessels that will not respond to further laser. Signs of new vessel activity include:

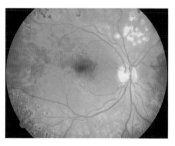

Fig. 8.18 PDR — post laser.

- neovascular buds to the new vessel bundles;
- tight networks of new vessels;
- a paucity of fibrous tissue.

Signs of inactive new vessels conversely include a general reduction in vascular calibre, both in the new vessels (Figs. 8.19 and 8.20) themselves and the neighbouring retinal vessels, and an increase in the fibrous component of the new vessels with an absence of budding tips.

Long-term results show that if a patient with 'high risk' characteristics responds well to scatter treatment, the chances are that the patient will continue to do well for at least the next 5–10 years. However the ETDRS showed that 11% of patients required vitrectomy with over prolonged follow-up. At 5 years, 2.1% of eyes that received early full scatter treatment and 4% of eyes that had treatment deferred required vitrectomy surgery (see Chapter 4).

Complications of PRP

Central visual acuity loss Laser burns disrupt the blood-retinal barrier allowing fluid to leak from the choroid into the neuro-sensory retina. This can result in temporary macular oedema with a corresponding decrease in vision. The blood-retinal barrier is usually restored after 7–10 days. However in the DRS following treatment, approximately 10% of

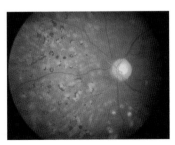

Fig. 8.19 Nasal fundal view of eye post PRP — note inferior venous beading and IRMA nasally near disc.

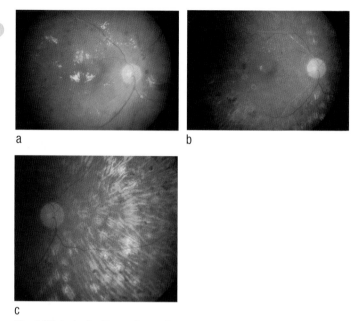

a   b

c

Fig. 8.20 (a,b,c) Pre and post laser views of patient with proliferative retinopathy and severe maculopathy — VA 6/24 at last follow-up.

patients had a one-line central acuity loss related to macular oedema exacerbation.

It is *more* common in patients with pre-existing macular oedema, and patients with maculopathy and mild PDR, that they should be treated with focal or grid last first followed by graduated PRP over two–three sessions to reduce the risk of this complication. Triamcinolone given via a posterior sub-Tenon's injection before PRP can also reduce the risk of maculopathy exacerbation in this situation.

Transient blurring of vision may also be caused by:

- induced mydriasis through the use of topical mydriatics agents;
- anterior chamber activity as a result of released pigment — rare;

- inflammatory response from repeated inadvertent iris trauma — rare.

Field loss In the authors' experience reduction in the field of vision to below that legally needed for driving is unusual with one session of PRP, but can occur after multiple fill-in treatments. It is obviously particularly important in patients who drive for a living, such as HGV drivers and taxi drivers. In these patients the risk of field loss should be discussed and may influence the distribution of the PRP and the spot size used. For example, in these patients it may be worthwhile using 200–300 micron spots for the posterior retina.

PRP burns can atrophy and coalesce with time and visual field defects may increase in extent.

Vitreous haemorrhage Vitreous haemorrhage, or the risk of further vitreous haemorrhage, is the reason the PRP is being performed in the first place and naturally a vitreous haemorrhage does occur occasionally after PRP. Again it is useful to discuss this with patients before doing the laser itself so the patients understand its significance and possible occurrence. Vitreous haemorrhage can limit laser treatment. If this occurs it is often possible to gradually fill in the PRP as the haemorrhage clears over several weeks. Diode laser can also be useful allowing better penetration through vitreous haemorrhage.

Glare Light sensitivity can be increased following PRP with dazzle and glare symptoms in bright sunlight. It appears to be a dose-related phenomenon and is more pronounced in patients with fair skin.

Impaired accommodation and pupillary abnormalities
Photocoagulation around the horizontal meridian can produce sufficient heat to damage the long ciliary nerves and therefore affect accommodation and pupillary reactions. This can also increase light sensitivity. Impaired accommodation can be bothersome for the first couple of weeks after a full PRP, but usually improves with time.

Impaired night vision and dark adaptation This can occur after extensive PRP secondary to a reduction in the number of rod photoreceptors with increasing scotopic thresholds and again may be relevant to discuss with patients, especially those with professions or hobbies requiring good night vision.

Colour vision This may also be affected following scatter PRP, where there may be general loss of hue discrimination. This may be related to direct cone destruction or due to a secondary effect from scatter or damage to the blue cone nerve fibres as a result of peripheral laser treatment. Infrared diode laser pan-retinal treatment is reported to cause less colour and contrast sensitivity loss compared with argon laser PRP.

Choroidal detachment This may be accompanied by a myopic shift of up to 4.0 D, with shallowing of the anterior chamber, and can occur after extensive full-scatter PRP. It is possible this may precipitate an attack of acute angle closure glaucoma. A choroidal detachment may last for several days and may respond to topical steroids and acetazolamide.

Asymmetrical retinopathy If retinopathy is very asymmetrical there are a number of explanations that could be considered:

1. Unilateral retinal veno-occlusive disease.
2. Unilateral carotid artery or ophthalmic artery stenosis.
3. The presence of a posterior vitreous detachment is relatively protective against neovascularization developing. Essentially new vessels need a vitreous scaffold to grow on which is why new vessels are uncommon after vitrectomy surgery. Patients with a PVD can however develop small abortive new vessels, often known as 'strawberries'. Patients with posterior vitreous detachments may never develop retinal new vessels but progress to develop rubeosis. This is particularly important to consider prior

to cataract surgery, and eyes with ischaemic retinus but no new vessels should be considered for "prophylactic" PRP in this situation.
4. Intraocular surgery can potentially exacerbate retinopathy.
5. Patients with glaucoma and retinitis pigmentosa have a low incidence of retinopathy from retinal atrophy.

Consent process prior to laser

It is important that patients undergoing laser for DR have a full discussion regarding the treatment so informed consent can be ensured. It is useful to cover a number of areas in the consent process:

1. Ideally arrange retinal photography immediately prior to laser, and explain to the patient, using the photographs, the problems they have. This often has a huge impact as the patients can actually see for themselves what is happening and can understand the risk to their vision. Explain to the patient basic retinal anatomy and what the likely natural history is in simple terms, such as if there are new vessels present these can bleed and if there are areas of exudation present how these can leak and affect their central vision.
2. Explain that laser has been shown to roughly double their chances of not losing vision from DR, both for maculopathy and proliferative retinopathy. However explain that it is not 100% effective and that vision can continue to worsen, despite laser treatment.
3. Explain that the aim is to reduce the threat to their vision by either reducing the amount of fluid leaking out of the blood vessels or reducing the size of the blood vessels that are growing if they have PDR.
4. Explain that constant follow-up and multiple treatments may be needed and that the laser is not a one-off treatment. For maculopathy explain that only affected areas away from the centre of the fovea can be treated, so that if blood vessels are affected in the centre these cannot be treated and the vision may get worse.

5. Discuss the possible risks of laser treatment including the possibility of vision getting worse. The depth of this discussion depends very much on the patients themselves. Some patients may choose not to discuss the risks whilst other patients may want a full and detailed discussion. For maculopathy the risks are certainly greater when treatment near the centre of the fovea is needed and clinicians should be careful to explain the risk of visual loss in these patients particularly.

6. Explain that the patient may notice small grey spots in their side vision for days to weeks after macular laser treatment, which usually gradually resolve with time.

7. Give the patient a brief description of the treatment. Explain that the cornea is 'numbed' with drops to allow a contact lens to be placed on the eye to focus the laser with. Tell them that when the lens is removed the eye can feel gritty and occasionally scratches can occur causing pain.

8. Explain that the laser is extremely bright and that when the contact lens is removed their vision will be completely black for a few seconds and then gradually return over several minutes. Also give the patient some idea of how many burns are likely to be applied.

9. After the laser treatment explain the importance of follow-up to assess whether they need further laser treatment or other interventions. If it is thought that they may have a high risk of requiring vitrectomy surgery then consider explaining the principles of this to them so that it can be understood that this is a part of the treatment in the same way as laser is. Vitrectomy surgery should not be viewed as a sign that laser treatment has completely failed. Instead it should be seen more as a part of an ongoing treatment plan.

Surgical management for DR

Vitrectomy surgery

The technique of using an automated cutting instrument to perform a pars plana vitrectomy was pioneered by an American

Ophthalmologist, Robert Machemer, back in the late 1960s and early 1970s. Since this time technological advances have led to its widespread use and improved outcomes with low complication rates.

Pars plana vitrectomy is a microsurgical procedure undertaken in PDR to:

- clear vitreous haemorrhage;
- relieve vitreo-retinal traction.

Vitrectomy instrumentation

Vitrectomy is performed using a range of instruments inserted through pars plana incisions i.e. sclerostomies into the eye which are positioned 3.0–3.5 mm posterior to the limbus in pseudophakic eyes and 3.5–4.0 mm in phakic eyes (Fig. 8.21). Most surgeons currently use 20 gauge-size incisions but smaller 23-g and 25-g systems are now available and increasingly used in selected cases. Typically three sclerotomies are required (Figs. 8.22 and 8.23):

Infusion cannula
In order to maintain IOP and transparency as blood-stained or fibrotic tissue is removed, balanced salt solution is infused into the eye via a sutured or self-retaining cannula typically placed in the infero-temporal quadrant of the eye.

Following placement of the infusion, a further two sclerotomies are made at the 10 o'clock and 2 o'clock positions in order to insert the other probes required.

Vitrectomy probe — vitreous 'cutter'
This probe contains within it a guillotine or oscillating-type vitreous cutter which can oscillate up to 2500 times per minute (Fig. 8.24). These can either be externally driven with compressed air or electronically within the hand piece. An aspiration line connected to the vitrectomy probe enables cut vitreous to be removed from the eye. Vitreous is therefore cut then aspirated from the eye minimizing retinal traction.

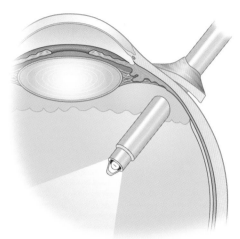

Fig. 8.21
Instruments pass through sclerotomies and enter the vitreous cavity through the pars plana, anterior to the ora serrata.

Intraocular illumination
Another instrument is inserted through the pars plana that contains a fibre optic cable attached to a halogen or xenon light source. This illuminates the inside of the eye during the surgery. Infusion lines can also be illuminated with narrow gauge light sources.

Accessory instruments
These include scissors (for dissecting fibrotic tissue), forceps (for peeling fibrous tissue), endo-laser probes (for intraocular laser delivery) and intraocular bipolar instruments (for haemostasis) (Fig. 8.25).

Viewing systems
A variety of intraocular viewing systems are in use. Hand-held irrigating contact lenses were first used followed by self-retaining non-irrigating systems. Increasingly however wide-angle

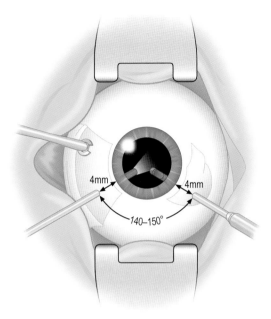

Fig. 8.22 Instrument set up for three port pars plana vitrectomy in phakic eye.

non-contact systems (e.g. the 'Eibos' or 'Biom' systems) with an image inverter system are being used because of the wide field of view obtained and the lack of need for a trained and observant assistant to keep the contact lens in the correct position (Figs. 8.26 and 8.27).

Anaesthesia

Vitrectomy surgery can be performed under either a local anaesthetic or a general anaesthetic. Patients with PDR frequently have significant systemic medical problems, notably ischaemic heart disease, cerebrovascular disease, anaemia, renal failure and hypertension, making general anaesthesia hazardous.

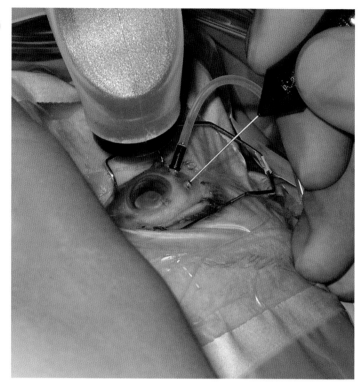

Fig. 8.23 Set up for vitrectomy — 25-gauge with guarded sclerotomies in this case.

Indications for vitrectomy surgery in proliferative DR

Vitrectomy surgery in diabetics is performed to treat the complications of neovascularization which are typically related to the action of vitreous contraction on the new vessels themselves. New vessels on their own rarely affect vision directly unless they are growing directly over the fovea and visual loss usually relates to vitreo-retinal tractional forces on new vessels, which can

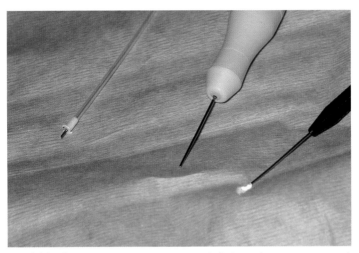

Fig. 8.24 Basic vitrectomy equipment — infusions, vitreous cutters and light pipe.

either lead to vitreous haemorrhage or retinal traction. Therefore a spontaneous complete posterior vitreous detachment is an excellent prognostic sign for patients with PDR, but unfortunately is uncommon. A developing posterior vitreous detachment with vitreo-retinal adhesions is the most problematical time for patients with PDR and is more likely to cause problems if new vessels are still active and densely vascularized (Fig. 8.28).

The indications for vitrectomy surgery include the following:

1. Severe vitreous haemorrhage from new vessels. Many haemorrhages clear spontaneously but some do not and these require surgery. The time most surgeons wait before intervening depends on a number of factors, but in general this time is getting shorter because of improving instrumentation, knowledge, techniques and results. Vitrectomy is done *early* if PRP cannot be applied (especially if there is rubeosis present) and vitreous traction is threatening the macula (especially common in type 1 diabetics) or *later* if a full PRP has been given and there is no risk of macular traction. Obviously a

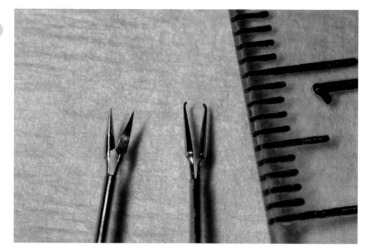

a

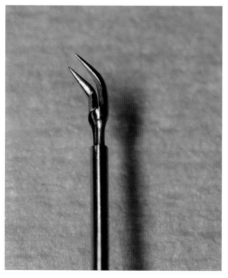

b

Fig. 8.25 *(a)* Vitrectomy scissors and forceps. *(b)* Horizontal scissors.

number of social and patient-specific considerations are important to the timing of surgery such as: only eye, previous complications, visual needs, home circumstances, general health etc. Recurrent, even light, vitreous haemorrhage can also be an indication for surgery if causing significant functional impairment — so called 'nuisance bleeds'.

2. Fibrovascular proliferation causing tractional retinal detachment involving, threatening or obscuring the macula (Fig. 8.28). This must be treated without delay although extra-macular tractional detachments may be safely observed, as they may remain stable for long periods of time. Surgery for diabetic detachment is more complex than for vitreous haemorrhage alone. This is because of the difficulty in relieving traction caused by fibrovascular membranes. Such membranes are attached to the underlying retina by vascular 'pegs' and attempts to merely peel off the membrane may cause tearing of the pegs, further bleeding and potential retinal tearing. (Fig. 8.29)

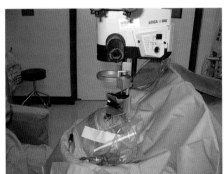

Fig. 8.26 Set up for three port pars plana vitrectomy (25 g in this case) — note indirect viewing system attached to bottom of microscope.

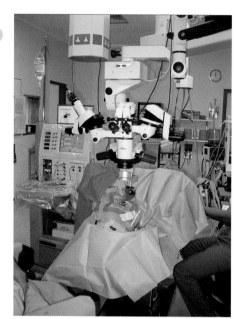

Fig. 8.27 Set up for three port pars plana vitrectomy (25 g in this case) — note indirect viewing system and vitrectomy machine on left.

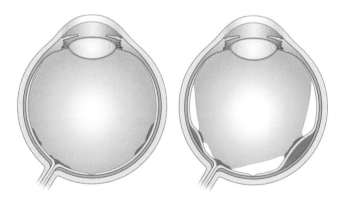

Fig. 8.28 Illustration on left shows new vessels with attached vitreous — no sequelae. On right the vitreous is starting to detach from the retina causing traction on the new vessels and resulting in vitreous haemorrhage and traction retinal detachment.

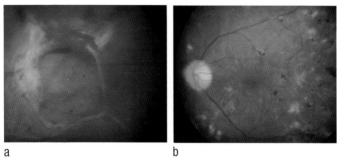

a   b

Fig. 8.29 (a,b)   Pre and post vitrectomy for vitreous haemorrhage and traction retinal detachment.
VA postoperatively 6/12.

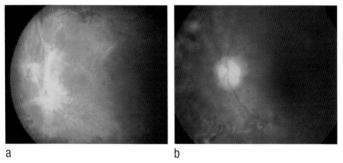

a   b

Fig. 8.30 (a,b)   Pre and 2 weeks post vitrectomy for dense fibrovascular membrane obscuring the fovea.
VA postoperatively 6/12.

3. Very severe fibrovascular proliferation after PRP (Fig. 8.30) even if vision is still good (opinion and practice varies between surgeons).
4. Combined tractional and rhegmatogenous retinal detachment should be treated urgently. This is because sub-retinal fluid may spread rapidly, involving the macula,

leading to irretrievable visual loss despite later successful reattachment surgery. Foveae affected by DR seem to be particularly at risk of deterioration after detachment presumably related to their relative reliance on choroidal blood supply.

5. Dense persistent pre-macular haemorrhage is often an indication for early vitrectomy as if left untreated the posterior hyaloid face may serve as a scaffold for subsequent fibrovascular proliferation and contraction and consequent tangential retinal traction giving rise to macular pucker or tractional macular detachment (Fig. 8.31).

6. Diabetic macular oedema with either visible vitreomacular traction including a thickened and taut posterior hyaloid face (Fig. 8.32) with tangential traction or occult vitreomacular

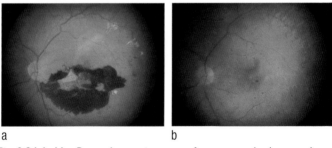

a   b

Fig. 8.31 (a,b)   Pre and post vitrectomy for pre-macular haemorrhage. VA postoperatively 6/9.

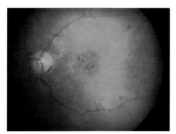

Fig. 8.32   Taut posterior hyaloid face with macular oedema.

traction on OCT. Clinical trials are also being carried out on the role of vitrectomy surgery for patients with macular oedema but no vascular membrane (VM) traction (see later).

7. Epiretinal membranes.

The aims of vitrectomy

The aims of vitrectomy include:

1. to clear media opacities such as vitreous haemorrhage;

2. to remove proliferative tissue causing tractional forces on the retina;

3. prevent further neovascularization by laser endo-photocoagulation and by removal of vitreous gel so removing the scaffold along which fibrovascular tissue can proliferate;

4. repair retinal detachment by excising tractional membranes and removing fibrovascular tissue from the surface of the retina.

Surgical technique

The central core vitreous gel is first removed with the vitrectomy probe. If there is no posterior vitreous separation then this is next elevated in an accessible area without tight vitreo-retinal adhesion. The optic disc is often a good location for this if no posterior vitreous separation exists elsewhere. The neovascular membrane complexes are now dissected away from the retina being careful to ensure that the dissection is in the correct plane and not in a false plane of vitreo-schisis, which can occur in PDR. This can be achieved using an 'en-bloc' dissection then delamination technique using the remaining posterior hyaloid face to exert antero-posterior traction to open up the plane of dissection (Fig. 8.33). Alternatively via circumcision from the posterior hyaloid face and then segmentation of neovascular complexes followed by their delamination from the surface of the retina. 'En-bloc' dissection and delamination involve the use of horizontal cutting scissors to cut through vascular 'pegs' joining the membrane complexes to the retina (Fig. 8.34). Segmentation may involve vertical cutting scissors to divide membranes between pegs in order to relieve traction between these.

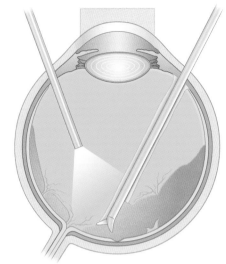

Fig. 8.33 Schematic diagram illustrating technique of en-bloc dissection using a-p traction of dissected free posterior hyaloid face to assist delamination.

Once the traction has been relieved the retina is carefully inspected for signs of retinal breaks. If identified these are treated with laser to form a surrounding chorioretinal adhesion and then gas or oil is used as tamponade. PRP is completed if deficient using indirect or endolaser and often continued up to the pars plana, which possibly reduces the rate of post vitrectomy bleeding.

Surgery can take anywhere from 30 minutes to 3–4 hours depending on the complexity of the dissection required.

Complications
Like any surgical procedure, vitrectomy is not without its potential complications:

1. Post-vitrectomy vitreous cavity haemorrhage can occur in some patients. This has a variable occurrence and it occurs in

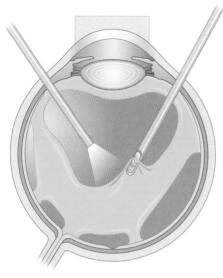

a

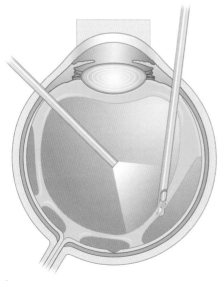

b

Fig. 8.34 Schematic diagrams illustrating technique of:

a. Core vitrectomy. (continued)

b. Circumcision of posterior neovascular complexes. (continued)

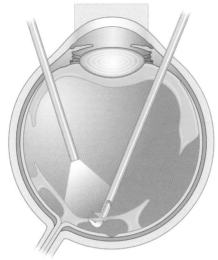

c

c. Segmentation of
   individual areas of
   vitreo-retinal
   attachments.
   (continued)

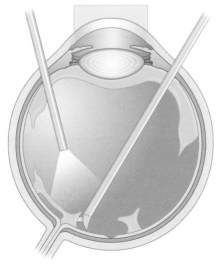

d

d. Delamination of
   membranes.

approximately 10–20% of patients following vitrectomy surgery. Anecdotally it is especially common in patients with very severe and active retinopathy at the time of surgery. Bleeding can occur immediately postoperatively or several months post surgery from ischaemically driven entry site neovascularization. Most cases are mild and spontaneously clear with observation as there is no longer vitreous present to retain the blood. However vitreous cavity washout is needed in 5–10% of cases.

2. Retinal tears and holes may develop which can be associated with instrument transit through the sclerotomies, related to posterior vitreous detachment generation or iatrogenic from instrument and tissue trauma during, dissection. If identified at the time of the procedure these can be dealt with using, e.g. laser retinopexy and gas injection. Sometimes these develop postoperatively and give rise to retinal detachment. Retinal detachment following vitrectomy is rare, occurring in less than 1% of patients.

3. Raised IOP following vitrectomy may be caused by a number of factors including:

- rubeotic vessel occlusion of the trabecular meshwork;
- over-expansion of intraocular gas used as a tamponade in the first few postoperative days;
- ghost cell ('old' red blood cells) or steroid-induced glaucoma;
- silicone oil-induced glaucoma caused by oil entering the anterior chamber or blocking the pupil;
- late silicone oil-induced glaucoma due to blockage of the trabecular meshwork by emulsified oil in the anterior chamber.

4. Cataracts can develop following vitrectomy surgery, especially in patients over 60 years old. Interestingly, in younger patients diabetes appears to be actually slightly protective for the development of cataract after vitrectomy.

5. Corneal epithelial problems related to diabetic corneal disease used to be a problem following surgery but are rarer now because of non-contact vitrectomy viewing systems.

6. Similarly rubeosis used to be a common anterior segment complication resulting in failure. Nowadays this is rare following vitrectomy surgery because of the ability to undertake perioperative laser.

7. The procedure carries the same risks as any other invasive intraocular procedure, namely endophthalmitis and choroidal haemorrhages, and these occur at an incidence of approximately 1 in 600.

Visual prognosis post vitrectomy

This will depend on the specific indications for surgery and the complexity of pre-existing vitreo-retinal abnormalities. Overall, about 70–90% of patients will get an improvement in vision with vitrectomy surgery with the final acuity result depending largely on the degree of maculopathy. Less than 5% may be made worse. As with laser treatment, retinopathy appears to go into an inactive stable phase after surgery and follow-up of patients in the ETDRS has shown that, once progression has stopped, patients with maculopathy, PDR and vitrectomy surgery (if needed) have stable acuities over 10+ years of follow-up. Certainly if an eye is doing well after 6 months, then the long-term outlook is generally good as the incidence of subsequent vision-threatening complications is low.

New treatments

Although retinal photocoagulation and vitrectomy are effective treatments for DR they do not address the fundamental disease processes associated with the occurrence of retinopathy. Furthermore laser is relatively ineffective at reversing visual loss. In the EDTR study only 17% of patients had any degree of improved vision following laser and only 3% improved by 3 or more lines. Many patients continue to lose vision despite laser and it is a destructive treatment with potential side effects.

There are a number of new treatments being developed for DR and this is a particularly exciting area at present. New treatment areas will be discussed in three main subject areas, namely new medical treatments, new laser technologies and new surgical approaches.

New medical treatments

New medical treatments for DR should be additional to the best possible medical control and not a replacement. Ideally they should inhibit pathological processes leading to retinal changes at an early stage to prevent progression of retinopathy or even its onset. There area number of different pathophysiological mechanisms in DR, which combine to produce the two main features of retinopathy, namely:

1. increased vascular permeability which results in vascular leakage and the accumulation of extracellular fluid (oedema and exudate);
2. the occlusion of capillary beds causing retinal ischaemia, which leads to new vessel formation.

At a microscopic level there are certain characteristic findings, namely:

1. a thickened capillary basement membrane;
2. loss of capillary pericytes which are the supporting cells of capillary walls;
3. loss of capillary endothelial cells.

There have been several biochemical mechanisms identified which, probably in combination, produce the above structural changes. These pathophysiological changes are complex.

Hyperglycaemia would appear to be the primary pathological event. High glucose levels result in two other glycolytic pathways being activated, namely the polyol pathway resulting in sorbitol production and the diacylglycerol pathway. Hyperglycaemia also causes protein glycation resulting in the accumulation of advanced glycation end-products (AGEs). The accumulation of sorbitol and AGEs cause oncotic and osmotic stress on retinal capillaries resulting in damaged auto regulation, retinal hyperperfusion and resultant vascular damage with sheer stress, wall stretching and blood-ocular barrier breakdown.

Increased retinal blood flow increases the already hyperpermeable state of the retinal vessels. As retinal capillaries get more damaged, areas of retinal ischaemia develop and this hypoxic drive leads to further vascular dilatation and further vascular damage. There is also evidence that high circulating glucose levels on their own can cause apoptosis of retinal pericyte cells, especially if glucose levels are suddenly reduced.

Hyperglycaemia stimulates nitrous oxide production and causes changes in the angiotensin-renin system in the eye which again cause altered vascular auto regulation.

Diacylglycerol has an important role to play in activating protein kinase C (PKC), especially the beta isoform which is thought to play a pivotal role in the production of DR. PKC is activated and also results in the production of vascular endothelial growth factor (VEGF) (also known as vascular permeability factor). VEGF promotes both vascular leakage and neovascularization and indeed is 50 000 times more potent than histamine in producing vascular leakage. VEGF via a feedback loop stimulates further PKC production (Figs. 6.2 and 6.3).

Hyperglycaemia causes a number of abnormalities of haemostasis which include increased blood viscosity, increased platelet aggregation, increased leukocyte adhesion to retinal blood vessels and a decrease in red blood cell deformability, increasing the chances of vascular occlusion in the damaged vascular bed.

It is the increased vascular permeability and occlusion of capillaries that causes problems with central vision in maculopathy. Vascular occlusion also results in increased VEGF levels, which secondarily results in neovascularization in PDR.

Based on these complex pathophysiological pathways, including others not described above, a number of new experimental treatments have been evaluated, exerting their therapeutic effect via a variety of different mechanisms. Several of these agents are still being evaluated in clinical trials and have included direct and indirect growth factor modulation, extracellular matrix alteration, and alternative DR pathways including dyslipidaemia, hypoxia and sorbitol. Although all have theoretical potential value, none has proven value as yet.

Direct growth factor modulators

VEGF is produced by the pigment epithelial cells, pericytes and endothelial cells of the retina in response to hypoxia from capillary loss and/or microaneurysm formation. Intravitreal VEGF has been shown to increase in concentration as DR progresses from non-proliferative to active PDR. It has also been demonstrated that argon laser PRP can reduce VEGF levels by as much as 75% in patients treated because of their neovacularization. This suggests that direct inhibition of VEGF activity may prevent neovascularization and other associated blood flow abnormalities. Consequently this has led to the development of a range of anti-VEGF agents. Clinical trials are currently underway that are investigating the use of various VEGF inhibitors. These include intravitreally administered pegaptanib sodium, which blocks the 165 isoform of VEGF (Macugen, Eyetech Pharmaceuticals, Inc, New York). Phase 2 trials involving 172 patients showed significant improvements in visual acuity and macular oedema in patients with foveolar oedema and phase 3 studies are now planned. Similarly trials using intravitreal ranibizumab (Lucentis, Genentech, Inc, South San Francisco, CA), a humanized anti-VEGF antibody fragment, which blocks all isoforms of VEGF, are underway. Studies using the off-label use of bevacizumab (Avastin, licensed for the treatment of colorectal cancer, Genentech, Inc, South San Francisco, CA), the parent VEGF antibody of ranibizumab, are also being carried out with early signs of efficacy in treating macular oedema, as well as retinal and iris new vessels.

PKC inhibitors. Various studies have demonstrated that when vascular tissues are exposed to increased glucose levels, PKC causes an increase in levels of diacylglycerol (DAG), an endogenous activator of PKC. PKC activity is increased when endothelial cells are exposed to oxidative stress, which is another cause of the development and progression of microvascular complications seen in DR. PKC comes in various isoforms, but the beta and delta are the most significant. PKC beta helps regulate endothelial cell permeability, blood flow and angiogenesis as a signalling component for VEGF. Increased levels of PKC beta have also been linked with increased leukocyte-endothelial cell adhesion and capillary occlusion.

Recent human placebo-controlled trials of the use of an orally administered PKC inhibitor called PKC412 have found that this can reduce retinal thickness substantially and improve visual acuity; however this drug was found to have disabling side effects.

Other randomized case control trials are currently underway which also include investigation of the use of the orally administered specific PKC B1 and B2 inhibitor ruboxistaurin mesylate, also known as LY333531. In animal models this has been shown to reverse microvascular complications of diabetes and prevent neovascularization. Results so far have indicated that LY333531 is well tolerated in patients with early DR and does reverse retinal blood flow abnormalities. Recently reported phase three studies involving 685 patients with moderately severe to very severe NPDR have shown a significant reduction in the risk of visual loss in patients treated with LY333531 as compared to placebo, although no differences were observed in retinopathy grade progression.

Pigment endothelium-derived factor (PEDF) inducers. PEDF is an endogenous inhibitor of angiogenesis and is thought to work by causing endothelial cell apoptosis (programmed cell death). Studies investigating PEDF have given conflicting results with some reports finding reduced levels of PEDF with retinal hypoxia as VEFG levels increase. In contrast other reports have found PEDF to be raised in PDR. Further studies are therefore needed to clarify the role of PEDF in the angiogenesis cascade. In the future PEDF may prove to be a useful intervention in the treatment and prevention of DR.

Indirect growth factor modulators

Somatostatin

Growth hormone, which is secreted from the anterior pituitary, has been linked to the progression of DR. Somatostatin is an endogenous growth-hormone-releasing inhibitor from the hypothalamus. Various trials have recently investigated the use of somatostatin analogues in patients with severe NPDR or early PDR. Octreotide is a somatostatin analogue and growth hormone/insulin-like growth factor-1 antagonist which can be administered by intramuscular injection. Early indications are that somatostatin may be effective at reducing the need for photocoagulation compared to a control group receiving conventional treatment. Pegvisomant is another GH-receptor antagonist which has been investigated recently but its effects on preventing DR progression have so far been disappointing.

Interferon alpha 2a

Interferon alpha is a peptide that influences gene expression and protein synthesis. It may have angiostatic properties by causing an inhibitory effect on vascular endothelial cell proliferation and migration. Interferon alpha 2a has been shown to be beneficial in certain types of age-related macular degeneration treatments by reducing sub-foveal choroidal neovascular membranes (CNV), in lesions not treatable with laser therapy. Preliminary indications suggest that alpha-interferon may also be useful in preventing the progression of neovascularization in DR. Excessive tiredness however was a major side effect in most patients treated. Further clinical trials are underway.

COX-2 inhibitors

Cyclooxygenase (COX)-2 is an enzyme that causes angiogenesis through prostaglandin synthesis in response to inflammation. Recently COX-2 was found in elevated levels in nerve fibre layer astrocytes of post-mortem patients with PDR. By inhibiting the action of COX-2, this may prevent progression of PDR. A human trial is currently underway which is investigating the efficacy of a COX-2 inhibitor, celecoxib (Celebrex, Pfizer, New York), on PDR.

Angiotensin converting enzyme inhibitors/angiotensin II receptor blockers

Angiotensin converting enzyme (ACE) inhibitors are frequently used as a method of anti-hypertensive treatment in diabetics. There is now fresh evidence to suggest that inhibitors of the renin-angiotensin system (RAS), i.e. ACE inhibitors, and angiotensin II receptor blockers (ARB), e.g. candesartan, may have beneficial effects on DR which are independent of their hypotensive properties. However these findings remain controversial as several other previous clinical studies (e.g. Heart Outcomes Prevention Study — HOPE, ABCD, UKPDS) have failed to demonstrate any beneficial effects of ACE inhibitors on DR.

Anti-oxidants
Diabetes mellitus may cause reactive oxygen species (ROS) production through glucose oxidation, increased flux through the polyol pathway and increased protein glycosylation. ROS may activate aldose reductase and PKC and increase AGE and DAG formation. In addition ROS stimulates VEGF production. Inhibition of ROS production can effectively block sorbitol accumulation, AGE formation and PKC activation. Vitamins A and E and pine resin extracts have all been evaluated for their potential use in DR treatment but with no convincing proven beneficial effect as yet.

AGE inhibitors
In the presence of hyperglycaemia, carbohydrates interact with protein side chains giving rise to the formation of Amadori products. These products are formed non-enzymatically via a series of intermediate steps. Such products then undergo a series of changes resulting in AGEs. AGEs are resistant to degradation and continue to accumulate indefinitely on long-lived proteins. These have been linked to the microvascular changes seen in DR, in particular capillary basement membrane thickening. AGE formation within the endothelial cell basement membrane inactivates endothelial-derived nitric oxide, which acts on peri-vascular smooth muscle causing vasodilation. This may result in impaired blood flow. Several cells, including vascular endothelial cells, possess receptors for AGE. Binding of AGE to endothelial receptors (in particular AGE-specific receptor — AGER) may perpetuate a pro-inflammatory signalling process and a pro-atherosclerotic state in vascular tissues.

AGE product accumulation in retinal capillaries, in animal studies at least, can be blocked by the use of AGE inhibitors such as aminoguanide. AGE inhibitors for the prevention of DR remains to be proven in humans.

Aspirin
Experimental results indicate that high-dose aspirin suppresses diabetes-induced retinal tumour necrosis factor expression and leukocyte cell adhesion molecule expression, which are implicated in endothelial cell injury and breakdown of the blood-retinal barrier. There is evidence that aspirin alone or in combination with dipyridamole could decrease the yearly increase in microaneurysms in patients with early DR. However in patients with mild to severe DR, aspirin therapy (650 mg per day) has been shown to have no real effect on DR progression. Aspirin may have beneficial effects in the early stages of DR but it may be that this is lost in the later stages of the disease.

Extracellular matrix modifiers
There is increasing evidence that microvascular changes may be partially caused by inflammatory processes. Evidence suggests that leukocytes can migrate and adhere to retinal capillary walls by adhesion between ICAM-1 on the endothelial cell walls and integrins on the leukocyte surface. Leukocyte migration into the neuro-sensory retina is associated with breakdown of the blood-retinal barrier, premature endothelial cell death and capillary ischaemia. All these changes occur prior to any fundoscopic changes. Certain integrins, e.g. 2vBeta3, can be identified in fibrovascular membranes of PDR and future clinical trials are planned to evaluate the effectiveness of certain integrin inhibitors.

Matrix metalloproteinase inhibitors
Matrix metalloproteinases (MMPs) are a group of endothelial peptidases that degrade extracellular matrix elements to allow migration of microvascular endothelial cells, which is an essential step in angiogenesis. Metalloproteinase inhibitors are being investigated for their safety and efficacy. AG3340 is a metalloproteinase inhibitor, which can be injected intravitreally

(Agourn Pharmaceuticals Inc, La Jolla, CA). An example of an orally administered metalloproteinase inhibitor which is under investigation is prinomastat. However results to date have been rather disappointing.

Statins: 3-hydroxy-3-methyl-glutaryl coenzyme A reductase inhibitors
Elevated serum lipid levels have been positively associated with hard exudates seen in DR and retinopathy grade. Anecdotally, it has been reported by a number of clinicians that early diabetic maculopathy which presents with just parafoveal streak exudates improves with the initiation of statin therapy and there is now evidence to support this. A recent prospective randomized study of 30 diabetic patients with macular oedema and dyslipidaemia found a statistically significant reduction in hard exudates versus controls after initiation of Atorvastatin, although visual acuity was not affected.

Oxygen
Recent studies have investigated the effects of directly treating diabetic retinal ischaemia with hyperbaric oxygen. These studies have generally reported improvements in visual acuity and reduction in foveal thickness. However much larger clinical trials are now required to investigate just how effective this novel treatment may be.

Aldose reductase inhibitors (ARIs)
Under normal conditions glucose is metabolized via the hexokinase pathway. In the presence of hyperglycaemia, high glucose levels saturate the hexokinase pathway and glucose is then metabolized by the polyol pathway. The polyol pathway converts hexose sugars such as glucose into sugar alcohols (polyols). For example glucose can be converted into sorbitol via the action of the enzyme aldose reductase, which is the rate-limiting enzyme for this pathway. Increased aldose reductase activity and accumulation of sorbitol have been found in diabetic animal models. As sorbitol does not easily dissolve across cell membranes this increases cellular osmolarity, ultimately leading to cell damage. Loss of pericytes in the earliest stages of DR

may be due to their sensitivity to polyols. Increased polyol pathway activity also alters the redox state of the pyridine nucleotides NADPH and NAD+, thus increasing their concentrations. Since these are important factors in many enzyme-catalysed reactions, many other metabolic pathways may be also affected. Consequently there have been attempts to target inhibition of the aldose reductase pathway with various ARIs but so far none have shown any clinical benefit.

Carbonic anhydrase inhibitors (CAIs)
Clinically and anecdotally CAIs such as acetazolamide can lead to a short-term improvement in macular oedema which may be useful as a temporizing measure in a variety of clinical scenarios. They are thought to exert their effect by their action on the Na/K pump in the RPE. Caution should be taken with long-term use because of the side effects of CAIs including electrolyte disorders and renal stones. Short-term side effects such as lethargy and a metallic taste in the mouth also limit their use.

Summary
As our understanding of the mechanisms that cause DR improve, more specific treatments will increasingly become available and many different products are currently under development. However many new pharmacological treatments which have been demonstrated in animal models have been shown to be less efficacious in human clinical trials. Ultimately normalization of glucose levels through better insulin therapy or pancreatic or islet cell transplants will be needed. For the time being however we will have to continue to rely on aggressive metabolic and blood pressure control in order to manage diabetes and argon laser as primary therapy for treating DR.

New laser technologies

The exact mode of action of argon laser treatment in DR is unclear. In focal laser treatment if there are discrete leaking areas these can be directly targeted with laser resulting in reduced leakage; however this is probably not the main effect of focal laser as laser is also effective in diffuse maculopathy when laser burns are applied in a grid or modified grid pattern to areas of thickening of the retina. There have been several theories on how laser exerts its therapeutic effect in this situation.

1. Laser-damaged pigment epithelial cells may regenerate creating a more effective blood-retinal barrier.
2. Destruction of retinal photoreceptor cells, the main consumers of oxygen within the neuro-retina, results in reduced hypoxia in the surrounding retina which in turn reduces the surrounding hypoperfusion and leakage.
3. Laser may cause the RPE to release growth factors and cytokines that restore the blood-retinal barrier.

Similarly the effect of laser on proliferative retinopathy is not known but again its effect may relate to:

- ablation of the highly metabolically active photoreceptor cells reducing surrounding ischaemia as above;
- stimulation of the RPE causing release of factors inhibiting new vessel growth.

Many researchers believe that laser probably works by its stimulatory action on the RPE. Argon laser, however, causes damage to all retinal layers including the choriocapillaris and the outer retina, and it is this destructive action, which causes most of the adverse side effects of traditional laser treatment. If a lesion could be produced on the RPE alone this could potentially still have a therapeutic effect whilst causing less tissue damage and less loss of visual function.

Diode laser with a wavelength of approximately 810 nm has a different absorption profile to argon laser at around 530 nm. Diode laser has less uptake by haemoglobin whilst maintaining a fairly high uptake in melanin, the principal pigment absorbing energy within the RPE. Modifications have been made to diode lasers to allow a micro pulse mode delivering the laser energy in very narrow pulses which can still produce a RPE burn whilst greatly reducing the surrounding spread of energy to neighbouring tissues. Trials have been carried out with micro pulse diode lasers using sub-threshold strategies; in other words producing retinal burns that are invisible when actually done but which produce a faint retinal pigment epithelial scar, visible mainly on angiography, several months afterwards.

Reports suggest that micro pulse diode laser seems to work but it is not yet in routine clinical practice. Some clinicians who have used the technique feel that it is not as effective as conventional argon and the results of randomized control trials are awaited. Treatment itself is also harder to perform, as it is not possible to see exactly which area has been treated, and so a rigid protocol of treatment application has to be adhered to. Also when performing argon laser the uptake of the argon laser is extremely variable in areas of oedematous retina. Without a visible burn being produced it is difficult to gauge the exact amount of laser needed in micro pulse diode strategies to produce any degree of RPE burn and both these factors may limit its introduction.

New surgical approaches

Vitrectomy

As mentioned previously, interest has recently been shown in the role of vitrectomy in the treatment of diffuse macular oedema which has been unresponsive to laser treatment. Interest was initially shown due to two observations. First, macular oedema appears to have a lower prevalence in those patients with an existing posterior vitreous detachment in DR. Second, macular oedema is actually fairly uncommon after vitrectomy for the complications of PDR and therefore the obvious question is, would an artificial induction of a posterior vitreous detachment with vitrectomy (or potentially in the future with a chemical vitrectomy with various proteolytic enzymes) improve macular oedema? Initially surgeons concentrated the technique on those patients with either macular pucker or vitreomacular traction or the small group of patients with a taught and attached posterior hyoid face over the macula. First impressions are that in these cases vitrectomy does help macular oedema.

The next question is whether vitrectomy works even if there is no vitreomacular traction present and if simply removing the vitreous from the eye improves macular oedema on its own. There are a number of possible theories why this may work in that it may increase oxygenation of the retina by allowing increased intraocular circulatory currents to occur and may reduce local concentrations of growth factors near the retina causing less vascular permeability. In some patients it clearly has a beneficial effect, but certainly in other patients it is less clear and the results of randomized control trials currently being carried out are awaited. Early results suggest that although there is a beneficial effect on macular oedema resolution, there is no significant improvement in vision compared to optimal laser treatment. Vitrectomy, however, may cause better long-term results, and further long-term controlled studies are awaited.

Intravitreal steroids in DR

Traditional methods of ocular corticosteroid delivery include topical, systemic and periocular administration. Topical steroid therapy is limited to only anterior segment diseases owing to the poor penetrance of steroids. Systemic administration allows drug delivery to the posterior segment, but long-term use leads to a range of unwanted side effects including, importantly, impaired glucose control in diabetic patients. Periocular injections, although systemically absorbed to some extent, appear to minimize most systemic effects; however the sclera and outer retinal barriers can impede drug delivery to their intended target tissues. Intravitreal injections enable delivery of therapeutically effective concentrations of steroids to the posterior segment, maximizing their anti-inflammatory and angiostatic effects, with no systemic absorption. Intravitreal triamcinolone has been used for several years in patients with uveitis and its role in the treatment of diffuse and cystic diabetic macular oedema is an area of interest at present.

Clinically, intravitreal steroids have also been shown to inhibit pre-retinal neovascularization in pig and rat models as well as decreasing vascular permeability and reducing macular oedema. In diffuse macular oedema there is widespread blood-ocular barrier breakdown and there is also increasing interest that microvascular changes in DR may be partially as a result of inflammation. Leukocytes and monocytes may play a role in capillary wall damage and occlusion. Leukocytes are thought to migrate and adhere to the retinal vasculature (on the endothelial layer) via cellular adhesion molecules such as intercellular adhesion molecule-1 (ICAM-1) and beta-integrins on the leukocytes. Other molecules also thought to be involved in this process include: vascular cell adhesion molecules, fibronectin and osteopontin. Leukocyte migration into the neural retina is associated with breakdown of the blood-retinal barrier, premature endothelial cell death and capillary ischaemia. All these changes occur before any lesions are observed clinically on the fundus. Evidence suggests that there is a link between inflammation encountered in DR with VEGF. VEGF is thought to produce inflammation by inducing ICAM-1 expression and leukocyte adhesion. When ICAM-1 activity is blocked, VEGF-induced blood-retinal barrier breakdown is suppressed. Similarly when VEGF is blocked, ICAM-1 up regulation, leukocyte adhesion and blood-retinal barrier breakdown are all reduced (see Chapter 6).

Intravitreal steroids probably work in treating diabetic macular oedema by a combination of several actions:

- Iinhibition of macrophages that release angiogenic growth factors;
- down-regulating MMP activation and preventing adhesion molecule expression;
- down-regulation of inflammatory cells and reduction in major histocompatibility complex (MHC)-II expression;
- down-regulation of ICAM-1 which mediates leukocyte adhesion and transmigration;
- effects on prostaglandin synthesis and the down regulation of VEGF.

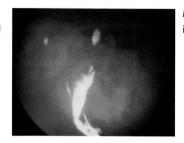

Fig. 8.35 Intravitreal triamcinolone injection.

They are given by intravitreal injection through the pars plana using a 27–30-gauge needle. Typically 4 mg of triamcinolone in 0.1 ml is given. It is white in appearance and after injection patients can notice visual floaters for several days to weeks (Fig. 8.35). Improvements in visual acuity of up to three lines have been reported and a reduction in macular thickness as measured by OCT by as much as 60%. As expected a common side effect of this treatment is raised IOP with most studies finding an increased IOP in 25–40% of patients. Similarly cataract formation is frequent, particularly after more than one injection. Posterior subcapsular cataract is most commonly seen.

Inflammation is another potential risk factor after intravitreal injection. Inflammation may manifest as pseudo-endophthalmitis (with the white triamcinolone appearing as a 'pseudohypopyon'), sterile inflammatory endophthalmitis or infectious endoph-thalmitis. True infectious endophthalmitis tends to present later than pseudo-endophthalmitis, perhaps 1 to 2 weeks after an injection, although patients may develop earlier signs that are masked by the presence of corticosteroids in the eye. The risk of endophthalmitis is reduced by using careful aseptic technique with the prophylactic use of povidone iodine.

Vitreous haemorrhage and retinal detachment are other potential hazards but very infrequently seen.

Unfortunately the effects only seem to last for up to approximately 6 months when re-injection is required. It is probably not practicable to suggest that patients should have repeat injections every 4 to 5 months. A number of slow-release preparations are thus being developed. Trials with fluocinolone acetonide implanted as an injectable pellet with an ethylvinyl and polyvinyl alcohol shell and others using a steroid combined with a degradable polymer, that results in gradual release of the steroid as the polymer undergoes hydrolysis, are being carried out.

Many clinicians only consider intravitreal triamcinolone in the following situations until more evidence becomes available:

1. Persistent macular oedema despite adequate laser treatment.
2. Persistent macular oedema (either unresponsive to treatment or non-treatable because view too poor) with cataract surgery.
3. Given prior to or concomitantly with laser in patients with gross macular oedema particularly if there is heavy exudate deposition at the fovea and/or multiple haemorrhages limiting laser treatment.
4. Where significant foveal oedema is present with high risk PDR requiring combined and immediate focal laser and PRP. Again if given, triamcinolone is usually combined with laser before or after injection.

Using current knowledge the following algorithm can be devised for treating patients with persisting foveal oedema despite laser treatment:

1. Obtain fluorescein angiogram to assess adequacy of treatment, the presence of other pathology and degree of ischaemia present: treat any untreated areas of diabetic-related leakage.
2. Careful medical assessment and treat systemic factors maximally.
3. Obtain OCT to assess presence of occult vitreomacular traction: consider vitrectomy if present.
4. Consider intravitreal triamcinolone (or new anti-VEGF treatments when available).

9
Co-existing eye disease with diabetic retinopathy

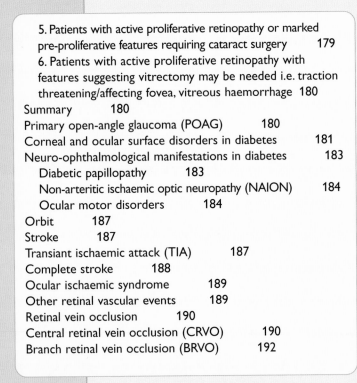

This chapter deals with some of the ocular diseases and conditions which can co-exist in patients with diabetic retinopathy. The appropriate management of cataract in diabetes is of great importance and is therefore considered in some detail here.

Cataract in diabetes

Diabetic retinopathy is the commonest cause of blindness in the working age group and diabetes itself is a common cause of cataracts (Fig. 9.1). In people with diabetes, cataracts and retinopathy are the most significant cause of visual impairment and blindness and people with diabetes are 25 times more likely than the general population to become blind. Diabetic patients develop cataracts more frequently than non-diabetic patients and at a younger age.

Diabetes is the commonest risk factor for cataracts in the developed world. There is a three- to fourfold increased prevalence in the under 65s and a twofold increased prevalence in the over 65s. It is actually the commonest cause of visual impairment in older diabetics with a 44% incidence of cataract surgery in the over 75s with diabetes. It has been estimated that somewhere between 10 and 20% of all cataract operations carried out in the UK are on diabetic patients.

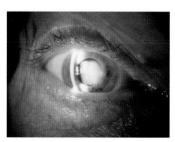

Fig. 9.1 Nuclear sclerotic cataract in a patient with diabetes demonstrating brunescence and white scatter.

Cataract in diabetics is significant for a number of reasons:

1. It impairs the recognition of site-threatening diabetic retinopathy (Fig. 9.2), both in the screening situation and in the detection of subtle macular oedema.
2. There is an increased surgical complication rate of cataract surgery in diabetics especially those with retinopathy.
3. There is a risk that retinopathy can deteriorate and that maculopathy in particular can be exacerbated by surgery.

It used to be said that because of the extra problems with cataract surgery in patients with diabetes, it should not be contemplated unless the vision was 6/36 or worse. However, this idea is outdated and perhaps the best time to undertake cataract surgery is simply when the patient is symptomatic and before the view of the fundus deteriorates to a significant level. Preferably this would be when there is no DR present as it has been shown that the severity of retinopathy at the time of cataract removal is the most important predictor of poor visual acuity. If retinopathy is present it should be optimally and maximally treated prior to surgery.

Surgical complications with an increased prevalence in diabetics

Modern cataract surgery using small incision phacoemulsification with secure predictable intracapsular intra-ocular lens (IOL) fixation has a lower rate of surgical-induced inflammation and

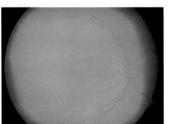

Fig. 9.2   Cataract obscuring fundal view with hidden occult central macular oedema.

loss of capsule integrity than previous techniques using extracapsular nucleus expression and intracapsular lens removal. This has greatly reduced the prevalence of surgical complications in diabetic patients but they can still occur and clinicians need to be aware of their potential occurrence.

Uveitis

This is more common in diabetics because of the increased levels of VEGF in diabetic eyes, especially in those with significant retinopathy (Fig. 9.3). Patients with poorer metabolic control and uncontrolled glucose levels also have increased VEGF levels. The more inflammation there is after diabetic cataract surgery, the greater the potential for retinopathy exacerbation to occur. Surgical trauma therefore should be kept to the absolute minimum.

Endophthalmitis

Diabetes is probably a risk factor for endophthalmitis (Fig. 9.3).

Posterior capsular opacity and anterior capsule phimosis

Both these are more common in diabetics, especially in patients with retinopathy. A large capsulorhexis just overlapping the optic edges should be performed and a large optic (6 mm or more) acrylic lens used.

Iris and irido-corneal angle rubeosis

This occurs secondary to the loss of the lens barrier and inflammation associated with surgery. It was far more common when intracapsular cataract surgery was performed and is more

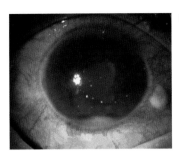

Fig. 9.3 Endophthalmitis.

likely to happen if capsule integrity is lost. Usually retinopathy has to be at least at the level of severe NPDR or PDR to put a patient at risk of experiencing this dreaded complication. Surgeons should be particularly wary of ischaemic eyes with very severe background retinopathy changes, but no new vessels in the presence of a posterior vitreous detachment. These eyes should be treated with PRP prior to surgery. Note that rubeosis can be very subtle and should be looked for carefully. (Fig. 9.4)

Progression of retinopathy

This is a disputed area with some studies finding no deterioration in retinopathy with surgery. However, there is other evidence that retinopathy progression can occur with cataract surgery, especially if complicated. One study showed a 74% rate of progression of retinopathy in operated eyes vs. 37% of non-operated eyes in the 6 months following surgery. Again it is especially common in eyes with severe pre-proliferative retinopathy or active proliferative retinopathy. Active retinopathy is also a very important determinate factor of visual outcome. In patients with quiescent proliferative retinopathy and no macular oedema, 57% in one study achieved 6/12 or better vs. 0% in patients with active proliferative retinopathy. Treated retinopathy is in general far more likely to have a successful outcome than untreated retinopathy at the time of surgery.

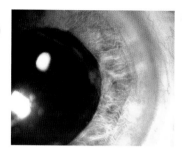

Fig. 9.4 Subtle iris rubeosis.

Laser immediately following cataract surgery can be difficult, because of:

- photophobia;
- diagnostic contact lens intolerance;
- poor mydriasis;
- IOL deposits and edge effects;
- posterior capsule opacity;
- vitreous haemorrhage etc.

Any laser treatment should therefore be undertaken prior to cataract surgery if at all possible.

Vitreous haemorrhage

This can occur following cataract surgery secondary to changes in the vitreous gel with increased vitreous syneresis following surgery. This is thought to lead to an earlier onset of posterior hyaloid separation from the retina and consequently vitreo-retinal traction on any new vessels present (Fig. 9.5).

Irvine Gass related cystoid macular oedema (IGCMO) and exacerbation of diabetic macular oedema

IGCMO is more common in patients with diabetes, especially if there is any retinopathy present (Fig. 9.6). There is probably also

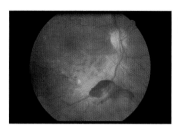

Fig. 9.5   NVD with a vitreous haemorrhage.

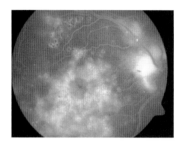

Fig. 9.6   Irvine Gass cystoid macular oedema (IGCMO).

occasionally true exacerbation of diabetic maculopathy with cataract surgery although this is partly secondary to IGCMO. Diabetic macular oedema can also be precipitated by cataract surgery and of course can be undiagnosed prior to cataract surgery, because of the cataract itself.

IGCMO is more common if there is diabetic retinopathy present and less likely to get better if there is retinopathy present. In patients with diabetic retinopathy approximately 50% get angiographic IGCMO and of these 50% spontaneously resolve by 6 months and 75% by 1 year. If there is no retinopathy present, probably less than 10–15% will develop angiographic cystoid macular oedema with corresponding levels of increased spontaneous resolution.

Diabetic maculopathy on its own is the main determinant of poor vision following cataract surgery in diabetic patients. It increases the risk of a visual acuity less than 6/12 sixfold.

If there is diabetic macular oedema present on day one after cataract surgery this is likely to be due to diabetes on its own, and studies have shown that this will not spontaneously improve in contra-distinction to IGCMO developing 1–2 weeks following surgery, which can, as discussed above, spontaneously improve.

Overall outcomes of surgery from published series

Where there is no retinopathy, or mild retinopathy before surgery, results are similar to non-diabetic patients, i.e. 85% obtain a Snellen visual acuity (VA) of 6/9 or better.

There is a poor prognosis in patients with non-proliferative diabetic retinopathy and macular oedema before cataract surgery, where retinopathy may progress in up to 50% of cases with worsening macular oedema. Focal laser for macular oedema prior to cataract surgery leads to less progression (no controlled studies) but 35–50% of eyes still require supplemental focal laser after surgery. A total of 40% of eyes with preoperative diabetic maculopathy who were treated with laser achieved 6/9 VA or better in a study by Dowler et al.

Proliferative diabetic retinopathy pre-cataract surgery is a risk factor for poor VA outcome. The prevalence of macular oedema is related to the overall severity of retinopathy, i.e. 3% for mild NPDR; 38% in moderate to severe NPDR; and 71% in PDR. There is also an increased risk of vitreous haemorrhage and retinal detachment and a higher risk of neovascular glaucoma than in NPDR.

In patients who have received previous PRP laser treatment, who subsequently undergo cataract surgery, 50% achieve VA of 6/9 or better overall. A total of 25% have a final VA of 6/60 or worse. Again the final visual outcome is influenced by the presence of preoperative macular oedema.

In patients with quiescent PDR who are undergoing cataract surgery, Snellen acuity of 6/9 or better is achieved in 60% of eyes without preoperative macular oedema. This reduces to 10% in eyes with preoperative macular oedema.

All the above points are important in the treatment and management of diabetic patients undergoing cataract surgery. The patient's general condition is obviously also important and glycaemic and hypertensive control should be optimized prior to surgery.

Ideally waiting lists for cataract surgery should be short. If this is not the case then diabetic patients should be re-assessed just prior to their surgery to ensure there has been no significant change in their retinopathy.

If the fundus cannot be visualized, then the history of visual decline and previous treatment is important. Pupil reflexes should be assessed to check for the presence of a relative afferent pupil defect (RAPD). A careful slit lamp examination is required in order to determine whether rubeosis is present. It may also be helpful to undertake an ultrasound scan to assess the anatomical state of the retina.

Risk of a poor outcome clearly varies with different levels of retinopathy and so the management of diabetic patients with cataracts will be discussed depending on the level of DR present:

1. Diabetic patients with no retinopathy

These patients can be treated as normal patients with cataract surgery. The only extra precaution that should be taken is that they should ideally perform surgery using a large optic acrylic lens with a large capsulorhexsis. The same postoperative regime can be used as with on any other cataract patient.

2. Patients with mild or moderate retinopathy with no macular oedema

These patients have an increased risk of IGCMO especially if there are peri-foveal avascular zone (FAZ) microaneurysms and haemorrhages. There is some rationale for giving all patients in this category topical steroids in addition to topical non-steroidals both four times a day following surgery as there is evidence for a synergistic effect of these two agents on the prevention and treatment of IGCMO. The author (D. Steele) also treats patients with **inactive treated retinopathy** in the same way.

3. Patients with macular oedema

In these patients if the view permits, their macular oedema should be treated maximally prior to cataract surgery with the aim being to dry the macula out before surgery. If their macula is dry by the time of the cataract surgery they then can be treated as in category two above.

If at the first postoperative visit (ideally within 5 days) the macula is oedematous then laser treatment should be carried out without delay and they may need fluorescein angiography before this. If the macula is dry at the first visit then the patient should be seen 2–4 weeks later. If at this visit they have macular oedema this is most likely to be IGCMO. Again angiography can be performed. Features to look for on this suggesting IGCMO as opposed to diabetic maculopathy are a hyper fluorescent disc and a petalloid pattern of macular oedema; unfortunately however these signs are not reliable. In this group of patients then one option is to increase the topical steroid and non-steroidals to 2-hourly and review 1–2 months later (if non-steroid responders).

If their macular oedema persists at this stage and the clinical impression is that it is mainly IGCMO then sub-Tenon's depo-steroid preparation can be given such as triamcinolone acetate 40 mg and again the clinical situation as regards the macula reviewed 4 weeks later.

If at this visit they still have macular oedema, then they could have the depo-steroid repeated and laser should be given to untreated areas of leakage identified on angiography.

4. Patients with macular oedema preoperatively who either have not responded to treatment or who cannot be treated because of the cataract density

In these patients the natural history and visual result with cataract surgery is often poor. One useful and convenient option is to combine the cataract surgery with intravitreal triamcinolone given at the same time. This has the convenience of one surgical procedure and is a theoretically optimal way of using triamcinolone for its short-term effect. There are concerns that combining the two procedures could increase the rate of postoperative endophthalmitis but this has not been the clinical experience. Usually the macula dries out very well following surgery. However even if the macula has dried out fully and if they have had no prior macular laser, then the patient should be carefully followed up and care given if macular oedema recurs.

5. Patients with active proliferative retinopathy or marked pre-proliferative features requiring cataract surgery

These patients should be treated maximally with PRP prior to cataract surgery. If PRP is not possible because of the density of the cataract then intra operative PRP should be considered. Intra operative PRP is most easily performed after irrigation/aspiration of cortex but before IOL insertion into the capsular bag. The capsular bag and anterior chamber should be filled completely with a viscoelastic substance prior to laser to allow safe indentation if needed. In the author's (D. Steel) experience indirect PRP is best undertaken using a 28-dioptre lens so that orientation regarding macular location is easier. Cataract surgery should also be performed using a sub-Tenon's block, as PRP in this situation is painful and if done under topical anaesthesia it will not be possible. A sterile indentor can be used to move the eye around and extra steroids should be given because of the blood-ocular barrier breakdown associated with PRP. Intravitreal triamcinolone can also be considered if there is frank macular oedema present. Alternatively sub-Tenon's triamcinolone 1 week prior to cataract surgery could be considered.

6. Patients with active proliferative retinopathy with features suggesting vitrectomy may be needed i.e. traction threatening/affecting fovea, vitreous haemorrhage

A combined cataract/vitrectomy surgery approach should be considered i.e. phacovitrectomy.

Summary

Cataract surgery in a diabetic patient is more problematic than in a non-diabetic patient. The severity and activity of retinopathy at the time of cataract surgery are probably the most important predictors of final visual acuity. Frequent follow-up is needed, far more than is needed for uncomplicated cataracts, and the patients and their relatives as well as other healthcare professionals involved should be fully informed of the difference between this type of cataract surgery and normal cataract surgery. In particular patients may get frustrated that the retina is being treated for no apparent gain before cataract surgery is undertaken and the reason for this should be carefully explained.

Primary open-angle glaucoma (POAG)

Open-angle glaucoma may be present especially if there is a family history of glaucoma in diabetic patients. The optic disc should be assessed (including disc photography) as in the non-diabetic patient with visual field and IOP monitoring (Fig. 9.7). The visual fields of diabetic patients who have had laser treatment, particularly if extensive, may be difficult to assess. Treatment of POAG in diabetic patients is similar to that in the non-diabetic patient.

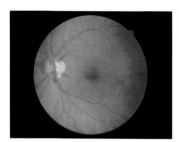

Fig. 9.7 Glaucoma. (Note 3 disc splinter haemorrhages.)

Corneal and ocular surface disorders in diabetes

Corneal sensitivity decreases with the duration of type 1 diabetes and is inversely correlated with the degree of neuropathy. A decrease in the number of long nerve fibre bundles imaged by in vivo confocal microscopy corresponds well with reduced corneal sensitivity. An increase in corneal thickness occurs in the early stages of the disease. Epithelial thickness decreases only in cases of severe neuropathy. Confocal microscopy seems to detect early phases of ocular neuropathy, since a reduction of the number of long nerve fibre bundles is detected earlier than a decrease in corneal mechanical sensitivity. In diabetics, confocal microscopy has demonstrated that corneal nerves are also more tortuous compared with non-diabetics.

Decreased corneal sensitivity and improper neural regulation in the diabetic cornea apparently leads to delayed epithelial wound healing and occurrence of recurrent erosions and persistent epithelial defects. Abnormalities of the epithelium and basement membrane may occur in diabetic patients with poor adhesiveness of corneal basement membrane complex with impaired hemidesmosome formation.

There is also an increased incidence of contact-lens-associated bacterial keratitis and neurotrophic ulcers in diabetics. This is mainly explained by an impaired immune response in diabetics leading to an increased susceptibility to infection.

Abnormally thick corneas have previously been reported in patients with diabetes and changes in corneal thickness have been correlated with severity of diabetic retinopathy. Studies have also shown that the light-scattering index of the basement membrane area correlates with the severity of retinopathy. Although the anterior stromal keratocytes are normal in most corneas there is evidence to suggest that anterior stroma could be altered in some patients with diabetes.

Measuring light scatter at the central cornea may reflect the changes in corneal thickness and hence the retinopathy. In one study a significant increase in corneal thickness was found in patients with background and proliferative retinopathy compared with non-diabetics. It has therefore been suggested that corneal light scatter could be used as a predictor for the progression of diabetic retinopathy. Light-backscatter analysis with optical coherence tomography (OCT) seems to be a promising emerging technique used for the objective estimation of corneal light-backscattering.

Dry eyes are up to 50% more common in diabetic patients compared with non-diabetics. Other conditions such as xanthelasmata, styes and blepharitis are also more common. Poor metabolic control and proliferative retinopathy are high risk factors for ocular surface disorders in type 2 diabetes and require careful follow-up.

Glycolacria is a term used to describe the presence of abnormally high concentrations of glucose in tears associated with hyperglycaemia. According to recent research undertaken in India, glucose levels in tears correlate well with blood sugar levels and can be used routinely in monitoring glycaemic control. Blood glucose levels were estimated quantitatively and also using glucose oxidase strips (Dextrostix). Tear glucose levels were estimated by placing a bent Dextrostix strip in the junction of the inner and middle third of the lower eyelid. Glucose levels in tears of 0 mg/dl, 25 mg/dl, 45 mg/dl, 90 mg/dl, 130 mg/dl, 175 mg/dl > 250 mg/dl were graded 0, 1+, 2+, 3+, 4+, 5+, 6+, respectively, using the Dextrostix strips. Oral glucose tolerance tests were also carried out in subjects. A total of 91.2% of patients with varying grades of hyperglycaemia recorded a positive colour response for glucose in tears. Correlation between blood sugar and tear glucose levels were also noted in the patients who were subjected to the glucose tolerance test. The concentration of glucose in tears changes proportionately with the blood glucose level. This method is very cheap and hence it has been recently suggested to have a role in community screening programmes for diabetes.

Neuro-ophthalmological manifestations in diabetes

Neuro-ophthalmological manifestations of diabetes mellitus may involve defects related to vascular, neuropathic or metabolic changes:

Diabetic papillopathy

In diabetic papillopathy (DP) there is a unilateral or sometimes bilateral transient swelling of the optic discs in patients with long-standing DM, but visual acuity remains relatively good (Fig. 9.8). Usually this condition resolves spontaneously over a period of several months. DP has been suggested to represent the extension of diabetic microangiography into the optic nerve head. It is important to differentiate DP from more serious disorders of the optic nerve head. In cases of bilateral optic nerve involvement, malignant hypertension and papilloedema must first be ruled out by measuring blood

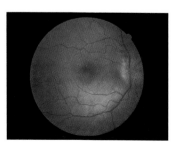

Fig. 9.8   Diabetic papillopathy.

pressure, undertaking neuro-imaging and then lumbar puncture, respectively.

True neovascularization of the disc also needs to be distinguished from DP by the orientation, the location of the vessels and the degree of leakage on fluorescein angiography. The teliangiectatic vessels of DP are arranged radially and lie within the substance of the disc. In rare cases, true new vessels at the disc (NVD) may be seen superimposed on DP.

Non-arteritic ischaemic optic neuropathy (NAION)

Non-arteritic ischaemic optic neuropathy (NAION) is a common cause of optic disc oedema, particularly in older patients. Risk factors for the development of NAION include ischaemic heart disease, hypercholesterolemia and DM. In patients with DM who develop NAION, this typically presents with quite profound sudden onset loss of vision, dyschromatopsia, optic disc oedema, moderate or marked relative afferent papillary defect and usually altitudinal visual field defects. Approximately 30–40% of patients with NAION improve spontaneously.

Ocular motor disorders

The most common neuro-ophthalmic manifestation of DM is diplopia, which most often results from ischaemia to the third, fourth or sixth nerves.

Sixth (VI) nerve palsy

The most common reason for a neuro-ophthalmological referral in a diabetic patient is ischaemic sixth (VI) nerve palsy. The nucleus of the sixth nerve (abducens) lies in the middle of the pons, inferior to the floor of the fourth ventricle. A VI nerve palsy presents with convergent strabismus and sudden onset horizontal diplopia. This diplopia can be minimized by turning the face into the field of action of the paralysed muscle, so that the eyes are turned away from the field of action of the paralysed muscle. Defective abduction is caused by weakness of the lateral rectus with normal adduction. The differential diagnosis of VI nerve palsy includes hypertension, compression (e.g. acoustic neuroma, nasopharyngeal tumour), trauma and ophthalmoplegic migraine. VI nerve palsy may also be a sign of raised intracranial pressure associated with posterior fossa tumours or benign intracranial hypertension. Hypertension is the commonest underlying association in diabetics.

An isolated VI nerve palsy is often due to focal small vessel occlusion with ischaemia of the VI nerve. Small brain stem infarctions are increasingly recognized as a cause of isolated ocular motor and vestibular nerve palsies in diabetic and/or hypertensive patients. Recovery with time is to be expected. However if there is failure to recover, then other investigations should be considered, e.g. neuro-imaging.

Third (III) nerve palsy

This usually presents with sudden onset diplopia; ptosis and pain may be present.

When a patient presents with isolated third (III) nerve palsy, the differential diagnosis is usually an ischaemic event or compression from an expanding aneurysm, which may rupture imminently causing mid brain haemorrhaging or tumour. It is always important to look for other cranial nerve involvement and to investigate these thoroughly. Blink reflex testing is sometimes a useful method for obtaining early diagnosis of cranial nerve compromise in diabetic patients who do not show any clinical symptoms or signs of CNS involvement.

Until proven otherwise, a III nerve palsy with pupillary involvement i.e. a dilated pupil, should be assumed to be caused by an intracranial aneurysm. This requires urgent management and neuro-surgical assessment including neuro-imaging, e.g. magnetic resonance imaging (MRI) and magnetic resonance angiography (MRA). It should also be remembered that anisocoria of approximately 1 mm is a fairly common condition and may be present in over 30% of these patients. This should be considered in the differential diagnosis in a patient with DM presenting with III nerve palsy. Anisocoria of greater than 2 mm should always be fully investigated using neuro-imaging.

Isolated III nerve palsy with pupil sparing is often due to microvascular disease (ischaemic III nerve palsy). Pupil sparing oculomotor palsy is possible in cases involving occlusion of the internal carotid artery extending from the bifurcation to the intracavernous portion, although not always. This still requires referral and very close observation. Again neuro-imaging is usually necessary if there is no improvement within a month.

Diabetic III nerve palsies may be caused by ischaemia in the mid brain or along the peripheral nerve. Most commonly however, the location of the ischaemia is peripheral rather than in the mid brain.

Although either DM or aneurysm is suspected in adults with oculomotor nerve palsy, young children with oculomotor palsy do not seem to have these entities. In children the most common causes of palsy are congenital, traumatic or neoplastic.

Fourth (IV) nerve pasly
This can occur in diabetes but is the least common.

Ocular motility defects
In addition to having cranial neuropathies, patients with DM may present with ocular motility defects from brain stem ischaemia. One such presentation is the 1–1/2 syndrome which involves horizontal gaze palsy in one direction and adduction deficit from internuclear ophthalmoplegia in the opposite direction.

Pupillary disorders
Pupillary involvement in DM most often presents with asymptomatic light-near dissociation with similarities to Adie tonic pupil, which is probably caused by neuropathy of the short ciliary nerve fibres. Pupillary hypersensitivity to pilocarpine is seen in tonic pupils and in some patients with oculomotor nerve palsy.

A less common manifestation of DM is Horner syndrome caused by autonomic neuropathy.

Orbit

Where DM patients present with thyroid eye disease as well, an increasing trend is now to opt for surgery rather than steroid therapy. However the surgical outcomes in DM patients are often worse than in non-diabetic patients. Radiation therapy is another option, but DR increases the risk of radiation retinopathy development.

There are a number of other orbital abnormalities seen with DM. It has been suggested that diabetic patients presenting with an acute orbital syndrome must be treated with a high index of suspicion of mucormycosis because of the rapid progression of the disease and its arterial invasion, necrosis and high mortality rate. Correction of acidosis is also important.

Stroke

Stroke is two to five times more common in diabetics compared with non-diabetics and is the third commonest cause of death in developed countries. Stroke is defined as the clinical syndrome of rapid onset of cerebral deficit (usually focal) lasting more than 24 hours or leading to death with no other apparent cause other than a vascular one. The various types of stroke are:

- **completed stroke** where the deficit has become maximal in 6 hours;
- **stroke in evolution** where the condition progresses over 24 hours;
- **minor stroke** where patients recover without significant deficit, usually within a week.

Transiant ischaemic attack (TIA)

Transient ischaemic attack (TIA). This refers to a focal deficit, such as weak limb, aphasia, or loss of vision lasting a few seconds to several hours, but where there is *complete* recovery. TIAs are usually sudden and have a tendency to recur and may herald the onset of thromboembolic stroke.

Complete stroke

The mechanisms involved are usually one of the following:

- arterial embolism from a distant site (usually the carotid, vertebral or basilar arteries) and subsequent infarction;
- arterial thrombosis causing occlusion in atheromatous carotid, vertebral or cerebral artery with subsequent brain infarction;
- haemorrhage into the brain (intra-cerebral or sub-arachnoid).

The most common stroke is caused by infarction in the internal capsule following thromboembolism in a middle cerebral artery branch. Lacunar strokes are a subtype of ischaemic strokes. In lacunar stroke, arterioles deep inside the brain become blocked and here lacunes are caused by occlusion of a single penetrating artery. The area rendered ischaemic takes the form of a small lacune or cavity, usually less than 15 mm in diameter. It all depends on exactly which brain structures are involved.
The deep penetrating arteries are small non-branching end arteries (usually smaller than 500 μm in diameter), which arise directly from much larger arteries, e.g. the middle cerebral artery, anterior choroidal artery, anterior cerebral artery, posterior cerebral artery, posterior communicating artery, cerebellar arteries and basilar artery. Their small size and proximal position predispose them to the development of microatheroma and lipohyalinosis. Although a lacunar stroke may be small, it can lead to major neurologic deficits, although most are less severe.
A much larger infarct may actually produce a less extensive (or intrusive) neurologic deficit for the patient. Hyperglycaemia in the setting of acute strokes correlates with poorer outcomes.
Transient neurological deficits have been associated with hypoglycaemia, which may be seen in children with type 1 diabetes. On administration of glucose, the prognosis is usually

very good and further investigation is not indicated. Acute hypoglycaemia also has a number of effects on vision which include blurred vision, impaired information processing and reduced contrast sensitivity.

Ocular ischaemic syndrome

Ocular ischaemic syndrome refers to the changes in the anterior and posterior segments of the eye that result from ischaemia, usually with carotid artery occlusion and poor collateral flow. Visual loss of varying degrees occurs and iris neovascularization is quite common. Most patients with ocular ischaemic syndrome have DM. Carotid reconstructive surgery has not been found to be helpful in recovering vision in ocular ischaemic syndrome.

Other ischaemic disorders are quite common in diabetics (see below). Where there is a component of vasospasm, this may be caused by the release of serotonin by platelet aggregation on atherosclerotic plaques. Changing a patient's diet from an artherogenic to a normal diet can reduce susceptibility to a vasospastic response to serotonin within a few months. It has been suggested that this may have therapeutic implications in the future with the development of serotonin antagonists.

Other retinal vascular events

Vascular events are common in diabetics (with or without retinopathy), including retinal artery occlusion, vein occlusion and ischaemic optic neuropathy.

Medical management in general includes the following:

- good metabolic control of diabetes including weight control, healthy diet and regular exercise;
- cessation of smoking;
- control of hypertension;
- prescribing statins for blood lipid control, e.g. Atorvastatin;
- cardiac problems, e.g. atrial fibrillation — consider electrocardiogram (ECG);

- exclude carotid disease — consider carotid Doppler scan;
- treatment of blood hyperviscosity if present, e.g. Aspirin;
- anti-platelet drugs, e.g. Aspirin;
- exclude temporal arteritis in ischaemic optic neuropathy or retinal arterial occlusion.

Retinal vein occlusion

All patients with retinal vein occlusions should have a thorough cardiovascular evaluation. The following investigations should now be conducted according to the Royal College of Ophthalmologists' recently published guidelines:

- full blood count (FBC);
- erythrocyte sedimentation rate (ESR);
- blood glucose;
- urea and electrolytes (U and Es);
- cholesterol;
- thyroid function tests (TFTs);
- protein electrophoresis;
- blood pressure;
- electrocardiogram (ECG).

Consideration should also be given to starting aspirin treatment.

Central retinal vein occlusion (CRVO)

Non-ischaemic CRVO is the most common type accounting for about 75% of all cases. It presents with a moderate loss of vision (Fig. 9.9). Mild to moderate retinal haemorrhages are seen distributed throughout all four quadrants but cotton wool spots are usually absent. Mild to moderate disc oedema and/or macular oedema may also be present. Fluorescein angiography may be helpful in certain cases. The prognosis is reasonably good in about 50% of cases with vision returning to normal or near normal. Cystoid macular oedema is the most common cause of reduced vision in such cases.

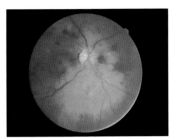

Fig. 9.9 Central retinal vein occlusion.

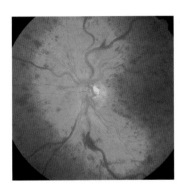

Fig. 9.10 Ischaemic CRVO.

Signs of ischaemic CRVO (Fig. 9.10) include very reduced vision, RAPD, a very haemorrhagic fundus appearance with cotton wool spots, retinal new vessels and there may even be vitreous haemorrhage. Ophthalmological management for ischaemic CRVO includes photocoagulation (PRP) to prevent or treat new vessel formation and neovascular glaucoma. Photocoagulation does not however alter the visual prognosis in CRVO and macular oedema.

Cydodiode laser may be given to treat raised IOP secondary to angle rubeosis.

Topical steroids and atropine may be indicated in order to help keep the eye comfortable in a patient with painful thrombolic glaucoma and a blind eye.

Branch retinal vein occlusion (BRVO)

Many patients with BRVOs do not require fluorescein angiograms, particularly on first presentation. Focal laser treatment may be helpful if there is macular oedema with unimpaired foveal perfusion after much of the retinal haemorrhage has settled. If the macula is ischaemic then laser treatment will not be beneficial. However sector retinal photocoagulation may be needed if there is widespread retinal ischaemia for NVD/NVE (Fig. 9.11).

Retinal emboli

Emboli are fairly common in DR and are often picked up during routine screening (Fig. 9.12). They appear as small white, grey or creamy spots, lumps or plaques within the retinal arterioles. There are three main types of retinal emboli, namely:

- cholesterol emboli;
- fibrinoplatelet emboli;
- calcific emboli.

They often appear at a junction or branch of the vessel and calcific emboli are the most likely to cause visual symptoms as they often block the central retinal artery near to the optic disc.

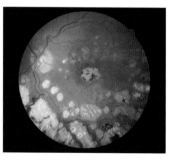

Fig. 9.11   Sector PRP for a branch retinal vein occlusion.

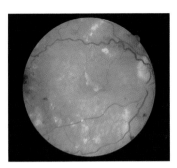

Fig. 9.12 Retinal embolus and NVEs.

The most common kind of embolus is a cholesterol embolus. They are usually easy to determine from a single exudate because they are present within the vessel rather than scattered throughout the retina. Many diabetic patients will have a raised cholesterol level and many will be on some form of statin and aspirin when they attend for screening. Cardiovascular evaluation and treatment should be carried out to reduce the risk of further cardiovascular events. Carotid ultrasonography should be considered to assess for significant carotid stenosis and possible surgery in symptomatic patients.

Retinal artery occlusion (central and branch)

There is usually a sudden painless loss of vision and giant cell arteritis (GCA) should always be considered in all cases of CRAO affecting older patients. Therefore an urgent ESR should be arranged, particularly if over the age of 65 years and if there are other typical symptoms of GCA. A general cardiovascular examination is required to exclude remedial cardiovascular risk factors such as atrial fibrillation, carotid bruits, heart murmurs and hypertension. If embolic disease is the cause then carotid ultrasound is indicated and possibly a cardiac echocardiogram. Other relevant investigations may include:

- FBC;
- glucose;
- fasting cholesterol;
- U and E;
- thrombophilia coagulation screening.

If the patient is a smoker they should be encouraged to stop and be referred, if appropriate, to their GP for smoking cessation advice and support.

If the BRAO/CRAO is within the last 24 hours, intravenous (IV) Diamox 500 mg may be administered in addition to ocular massage. Paracentesis of the anterior chamber may also be considered if symptoms are less than 12 hours' duration. If the sudden vision loss was more than 24 hours, then recovery of vision is very unlikely. Low dose aspirin is usually commenced.

Neovascular glaucoma (NVG)

In NVG elevation of IOP is caused by synechial angle closure through contraction of fibrovascular tissue. The common factor in all eyes with NVG is severe, diffuse and chronic retinal ischaemia. Ischaemic CRVO is the commonest cause, followed by patients with long-standing diabetes who also have proliferative DR. The risk of NVG is further increased by the following extracapsular cataract extraction (see cataract section).

Management of NVG in diabetes includes:

- argon laser PRP;
- if iris new vessels (NVIs) regress, but IOP is not controlled medically, then options include: 1) filtration surgery, often with the use of anti-metabolites such as 5-fluorouracil (5-FU) or Mitomycin C; 2) Cyclodiode laser; and 3) artificial drainage shunts such as Molteno or Ahmed valves;
- topical steroids, cycloplegics or occasionally enucleation may also be required to help relieve pain.

Ghost cell glaucoma in diabetes

This type of secondary glaucoma is associated with degenerated intraocular red blood cells that cause trabecular obstruction. It can occur after vitreous haemorrhage in any eye with communication between the vitreous and anterior segment with disruption of the anterior hyaloid face (especially in eyes already aphakic). After around 2 weeks in the vitreous, the haemoglobin leaks out of the red blood cells, turning them into degenerated 'ghost cells' which then pass through any defect in the anterior vitreous face into the anterior chamber, thus obstructing the trabecular meshwork.

Management:

1. topical anti-glaucoma agents, e.g. beta blockers and carbonic anhydrase inhibitors.
2. vitrectomy surgery.

Choroidal naevi

Choroidal naevi (Fig. 9.13) are fairly common occurring in approximately 5% of screened patients and are sub-retinal pigment patches found in the choroidal layer, usually flat, circular and greyish in appearance. They appear on screening as a dark shadow in the fundus, are usually fairly small and can have

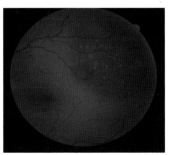

Fig. 9.13   Large naevus.

drusen over them. However naevi greater than 3–4 disc diameters in size should be considered for referral to evaluate any signs of choroidal melanoma. Due to the naevus being flat and sub-retinal, the retinal vessels should lie over the top of the naevus without any displacement. Should the vessels appear unusual and in particular look to be raised in any way then this may suggest possible malignancy and again referral is warranted for further detailed ophthalmological assessment.

Age-related macular degeneration

It is important to remember that diabetic patients are not immune from macular degeneration whether or not retinopathy is present. Distinguishing exudates (Fig. 9.14) from drusen (Fig. 9.15) can be challenging but the key differences are listed below (see Table 9.1).

The management of wet (exudative) macular degeneration is similar to that in the non-diabetic patient.

Epiretinal membrane at the macula

This may occur in diabetes with or without retinopathy. This is caused by contraction of fibrous tissue on the surface of macula, usually associated with the presence of a posterior vitreous

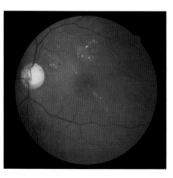

Fig. 9.14 Streak exudates.

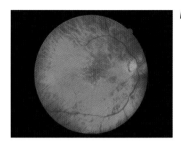

Fig. 9.15 Macular drusen.

Table 9.1 Distinguishing exudates from drusen

Exudates	Drusen
Other signs of DR especially microaneurysms	Deeper
Yellow hard appearance	Creamy/white
Streaks	Round
Circinate/semi-circinate pattern	Not typically circinate

detachment (PVD) (Fig. 9.16). Vision may be distorted in cellophane maculopathy and can be classified according to the severity of retinal distortion, associated slit-lamp biomicroscopic changes and associated ocular disorders. If symptomatic the patient may be a candidate for vitrectomy and membrane peel.

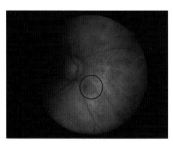

Fig. 9.16 Weiss ring after a PVD.

Chorio-retinal folds

Any condition causing a reduction in the area of inner surface of the sclera (scleral thickening or scleral shrinkage) will cause the inner portion of the choroid, including Bruch's membrane, the overlying retinal pigment epithelium (RPE) and the outer retinal layers, to be thrown into a series of folds or wrinkles.

These may appear as horizontal, vertical or oblique folds that are parallel in appearance (Fig. 9.17). On slit-lamp the crest (peak) of the fold appears yellow and the valley (trough) appears darker. These are often located supero-temporal and circumferential to the macula. If unilateral they can be associated with orbital masses. They can occur bilaterally in hypermetropes and may be asymptomatic. The management depends entirely on the presumed cause.

Myelinated nerve fibres

Myelination occurs when the myelin sheath of the optic nerve fibres extends through the laminar cribosa and is visible either adjacent to the optic nerve head or can follow the nerve fibre layer across the retina (Fig. 9.18). It is a congenital condition requiring no treatment. The patient's vision will be unaffected. On photography the myelinated nerve fibres reflect light brilliantly and appear as a bright white patch which can obscure vessels

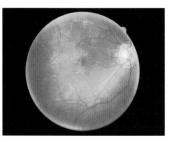

Fig. 9.17   Chorio-retinal folds.

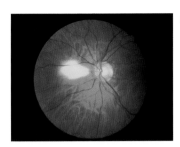

Fig. 9.18 Myelinated nerves.

emerging from the optic disc but are usually quite easy to determine from exudates or cotton wool spots. These may occur peripherally as well as giving a feathery white appearance in the nerve fibre layer.

Newborns of diabetic mothers

Optic nerve hypolasia (which may be unilateral or bilateral) has been reported in children of mothers with type 1 DM. Potential risk factors include: female sex, lower birth weight, shorter pregnancy and poorer control of the mother's DM. Newborns of mothers with type 1 DM or gestational diabetes have been found to have numerous iris abnormalities, including hypolasia of the iris stroma, significant tortuosity and dilatation of the iris vessels and a decreased response to dilation to tropicamide.

Asteroid hyalosis

Asteroid hyalosis comprises of lipid droplets suspended in the vitreous gel. If severe enough these can affect vision which in extreme cases may justify vitrectomy surgery. As far as screening for DR these can obscure the retinal image and make distinguishing exudates, if present, from asteroid quite difficult. The simplest way to distinguish between the two is to take a second photograph having asked the patient to move their eyes between shots. Asteroid will move position whereas exudates will remain in their fixed location on the retinal image (Fig. 9.19).

Unusual findings

Occasionally the strangest things can be detected on diabetic retinal screening. Fig. 9.20 is from a lady who attended for diabetic screening who had a history of ischaemic heart disease. Approximately 6 weeks before this photograph was taken she had undergone heart bypass surgery. Note the thin black line within the supero-temporal branch retinal artery. This was not an artefact but in fact was later confirmed to be a stitch remnant that had travelled up from the heart through the carotid artery and ophthalmic artery before becoming lodged in the retina at the arterial bifurcation. No significant effect was caused from this and the branch artery did not occlude.

Conclusions

While examining diabetics with retinopathy there is a wide variety of other medical retinal and anterior segment conditions that may give rise to the need for referral. However not all these conditions do actually need to be referred.

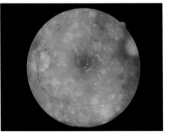

Fig. 9.19 Asteroid hyalosis.

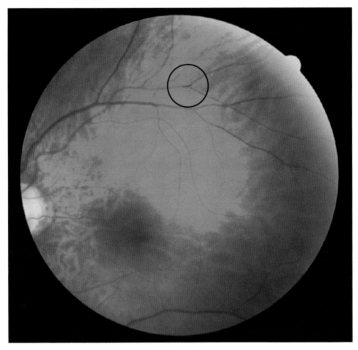

Fig. 9.20 Stitch remant lodged in supero-temporal retinal artery. The patient had undergone heart bypass surgery 6 weeks earlier.

Further reading

Chatterjee D 2003 Glucose levels in tears useful for monitoring diabetic control. *Journal of the Association of Physicians of India* **101**: 481–483

Jianhua W, Simpson T L, Fonn D 2004 Objective measurements of corneal light-backscatter during corneal swelling, by optical coherence tomography. *Investigative Ophthalmology and Visual Science* **45**: 3493–3498

Lattanzio R, Brancato R, Bandello F M et al 2001 Florid diabetic retinopathy (FDR): a long term follow-up study. *Graefes Archive for Clinical and Experimental Ophthalmology* **239**: 182–187

Mittra R A, Borrillo J L, Dev S et al 2000 Retinopathy progression and visual outcomes after phacoemulsification in patients with diabetes mellitus. *Archives of Ophthalmology* **118**: 912–917

Morishige N, Chikama T, Sassa Y et al 1999 Correlation of corneal light scattering index measured by a confocal microscope with stages of diabetic retinopathy. *Investigative Ophthalmology & Visual Science* **40(4)**: S620 Abstract no. 3261

Moster M L 1999 Neuro-ophthalmology of diabetes. *Current Opinions in Ophthalmology* **10**: 376–381

Nazliel B, Yetkin I, Irkec C et al 2001 Blink reflex abnormalities in diabetes mellitus. *Diabetes/Metabolism Research and Reviews* **17**: 396–400

Patel S V, Mutyala S, Leske D A 2004 Incidence, associations and evaluation of sixth nerve palsy using a population-based method. *Ophthalmology* **111**: 369–375

Recchia F M, Brown G C 2000 Systemic disorders associated with retinal vascular occlusion. *Current Opinion in Ophthalmology* **11**: 462–467

Sadiq S A, Sleep T, Amoaku W M 1999 The visual results and changes in retinopathy in diabetic patients following cataract surgery. *European Journal of Ophthalmology* **9**: 14–20

Sadun A A 1999 Neuro-ophthalmic manifestations of diabetes. *Ophthalmology* **106**: 1047–1048

Shukla D, Rajendran A, Singh J et al 2003 Atypical manifestations of diabetic retinopathy. *Current Opinion in Ophthalmology* **14**: 317–377

Squirrell D, Bhola R, Bush J et al 2002 A prospective, case controlled study of the natural history of diabetic retinopathy and maculopathy after uncomplicated phacoemulsification cataract surgery in patients with type 2 diabetes. *British Journal of Ophthalmology* **86**: 565–571

Thomke F, Gutmann L, Hopf H C 1999 Most diabetic third nerve palsies are peripheral. *Neurology* **11**: 894–895

Wipf J E, Pauuw D S 2000 Ophthalmologic emergencies in the patient with diabetes. *Endocrinology and Metabolism Clinics of North America* **29**: 813–829

10
Preventing diabetic retinopathy through control of systemic factors

Introduction

Risk factors that modify the rate of onset and progression of retinopathy or the development of visual loss due to diabetic retinopathy (DR) are numerous. The main risk factors appear to be duration of diabetes and blood glucose control. In addition to these, aggressive treatment of systemic conditions that exacerbate or accelerate the course of diabetic microvascular and macrovascular disease are also very important. These include elevated systolic blood pressure, urinary albumin excretion, hyperlipidaemia, smoking, increased body mass index, sleep apnoea and pregnancy. These will be discussed below.

Duration of diabetes

Duration of diabetes is defined for clinical purposes as the time from diagnosis of diabetes. However, it is recognized that sub-clinical diabetes may be present for a significant period prior to diagnosis.

There is a clear relationship between the duration of diabetes and the development of retinopathy in both type 1 and type 2 diabetics. This has been demonstrated for type 1 diabetes in the US Diabetes Control and Complications Trial (DCCT) and less clearly in the United Kingdom Prospective Diabetes Study (UKPDS) for type 2 diabetics. The duration of diabetes is a very important risk factor for the progression and severity of DR in type 1 and type 2 diabetics.

Hyperglycaemia

Prolonged exposure to hyperglycaemia causes microvascular complications, such as retinopathy, nephropathy, and neuropathy. Studies have demonstrated that hyperglycaemia predicts incidence and progression of DR. The DCCT and the UKPDS are two randomized clinical trials that have conclusively showed the efficacy of glycaemic control in preventing DR.

The DCCT study showed that intensive glycaemic control in type 1 diabetics with no baseline retinopathy or mild to moderate DR demonstrated a decrease in the rate of progression of retinopathy, the development of severe retinopathy, or the need for photocoagulation. The DCCT showed that intensive insulin therapy effectively delays the onset and slows the progression of DR in patients with type 1 diabetes. In the primary prevention cohort (those with no retinopathy at baseline), intensive therapy reduced the adjusted mean risk for the development of retinopathy by 76% compared with conventional therapy. In the secondary intervention cohort (those with mild retinopathy at baseline), intensive therapy slowed the progression of retinopathy by 54% and reduced the development of proliferative or severe non-proliferative retinopathy by 47%.

The epidemiology of diabetes interventions and complications (EDIC) research group followed patients for 4 years after the conclusion of the DCCT and found that the benefits of intensive diabetes control persisted even with increasing hyperglycaemia (HbA1C increased from 7.2 to 7.9%). The intensive glycaemic control group continued to demonstrate a decrease in retinopathy endpoints, including worsening retinopathy, proliferative DR, macular oedema and the need for laser treatment.

The UKPDS revealed that improved control in patients with type 2 diabetes not only led to a reduction in retinopathy but also reduced overall microvascular complications by 25%. A one-point decrease in HbA1C was associated with a 35% reduction in risk of microvascular complications. The American Diabetes Association advocates an HbA_{1C} goal of less than 7%.

Diet and exercise are also important factors in the care of a patient with diabetes. Exercise alone reduces the concentration of HbA1C by about 0.65 points and should be strongly encouraged. Risks of progressive nephropathy and neuropathy are also reduced with tight glucose control.

Intensive insulin therapy is associated with certain risks including more frequent hypoglycaemic episodes, increased wound infections and weight gain. Patients should be advised to keep glycaemic control as good as possible.

In patients with impaired glucose tolerance, the Hoorn study found that the prevalence of developing retinopathy was 13.6% in individuals with impaired glucose metabolism and 17.5% in individuals with newly diagnosed diabetes. The Hoorn study also showed that the prevalence of retinopathy increased as HbA1C increased.

Any reduction in HbA1C is beneficial in reducing the development of new and progression of existing DR. Patients should be aware of their HbA1C, what it means and how it can be lowered. Ideally patients should be encouraged to maintain their HbA1C below 5–6% and ideally 4–5%. Caution should be exercised where HbA1C is reduced too quickly as this can exacerbate temporary worsening of DR; however long-term benefits should be emphasized.

Hypertension

The regulation of blood flow within the retinal microvasculature is impaired in diabetes, leading to increased microvascular hypertension and to increased susceptibility to injury from even modest levels of systemic hypertension. Even relatively small increases in either systolic or diastolic blood pressure, that may be within the normal range for non-diabetic people, significantly increases the risk for the development and progression of DR compared with diabetic patients with lower blood pressures.

In multiple trials, aggressive blood pressure treatment has been accompanied by improved outcomes in retinopathy and nephropathy (see below) without an observed threshold blood pressure which was not beneficial. Both the American and British Diabetes societies now recommend that for both type 1 and type 2 diabetes, hypertension should be aggressively treated to levels less than 130 mmHg systolic and less than 80 mmHg diastolic and to less than 75 mmHg where there is any evidence of proteinuria (see below). These are also now recommended for any patients with DR. The blood pressure in diabetic patients is often labile with neurogenic orthostatic hypertension as well as nocturnal supine hypertension. Care should be taken to avoid attributing elevated blood pressure to white coat hypertension, as this may delay appropriate intervention. Twenty-four hour blood pressure monitoring is recommended for treatment decisions, aiming to control all blood pressure measurements (i.e. diastolic and systolic) to target levels. Interestingly nocturnal supine hypertension may account for some of the worsening vision patients often experience in the morning.

In both the Wisconsin Epidemiologic Study of Diabetic Retinopathy and the UKPDS, diabetic retinopathy progressed significantly more slowly with more tightly controlled blood pressure. Risks of progressive nephropathy and neuropathy are also reduced with good blood pressure control. At present there is also no definitive evidence suggesting there is any particular advantage of treating systolic versus diastolic blood pressure levels. This was certainly the findings of the Appropriate Blood Pressure Control in Diabetes (ABCD) trial where patients were randomized to either intensive or moderate blood pressure control. This showed that there was no difference between the intensive control group and the moderate control group in terms of progression of DR or nephropathy. However any reduction in blood pressure, especially systolic, is beneficial (<130 mmHg is the ideal target). Patients should be aware of their blood pressure and what they can do to lower it. This should be regularly monitored and patients should be fully aware of the consequences of not abiding to prescribed treatment regimens.

The UKPDS evaluated the effects of blood pressure and glycaemic control in the prevention and progression of DR in type 2 diabetes. Subjects were randomly assigned to two groups. The first group were assigned to intensive blood pressure control (<144/82). The second group was assigned to a less tightly controlled blood pressure (<154/87). There was a 34% reduction in the risk of DR progression and a 37% reduction in diabetic microvascular endpoints in the first group (intensive control).

In the UKPDS however, 29% of patients needed three or more antihypertensive drugs to reach the target blood pressure levels. At least 60% of patients needed two antihypertensive drugs after

9 years. In practice many patients need combinations of treatments from different drug classes to manage their hypertension and this should be aggressively pursued. The choice of antihypertensive agent for diabetics is still controversial, but include the following types:

- Diuretics are commonly prescribed and are relatively cheap which is an important factor in the current financial constraints of the Health Service. Diuretics however do slightly raise blood sugar levels, aggravate dyslipidaemia and at higher doses cause sexual dysfunction.
- Beta-blockers are also inexpensive and do significantly reduce risk of death and cardiac events after myocardial infarction (heart attack) as well as when used as primary prevention. However they do produce a range of unwanted side effects in many patients including reduced hypoglycaemic awareness, conduction disturbances and sexual dysfunction.
- Alpha-receptor antagonists, angiotensin converting enzyme (ACE) inhibitors and calcium channel blockers appear to have no adverse effects on glycaemic control and insulin resistance. Oedema and tachycardia limit the use of calcium channel blockers and an increased risk of adverse cardiovascular events has been shown with alpha-blockers versus diuretics and with calcium channel blockers versus ACE inhibitors in diabetic patients.

ACE inhibitors are commonly used in diabetics to manage blood pressure. Several studies have reported that the use of ACE inhibitors may have a protective effect against the progression and development of DR and slow the progression of nephropathy. This is because ACE inhibitors and angiotensin II receptor blockers cause dilation of efferent glomerular arterioles which produces a protective effect with respect to nephropathy. As a result of this these drugs are preferred in the early treatment of hypertension in diabetics with microalbuminuria.

ACE inhibitors however appear to be no more effective than beta-blockers in the treatment of moderate to severe DR in type 2 diabetics. In another recent study ACE inhibitors were found to decrease levels of vitreous vascular endothelial growth factor, possibly protecting against the development of proliferative DR.

The UKPDS also showed that there was no difference in the use of ACE inhibitors compared with beta-blockers with regards to the progression of DR in type 2 diabetics. This demonstrated that blood pressure control and not medication type is the most important factor. The ABCD trial was a prospective randomized trial comparing the effects of intensive and moderate blood pressure control in hypertensive type 2 diabetics. This study showed that there was no difference in the progression of retinopathy of patients assigned to calcium channel blockers compared to ACE inhibitors (enalapril).

The DIRECT study was a large randomized controlled clinical trial which further investigated the efficacy of ACE inhibitors in preventing the incidence and progression of retinopathy in type 1 and type 2 diabetics. This demonstrated very limited beneficial effect.

The EURODIAB Controlled Trial of Lisinopril in Insulin-Dependent Diabetes Mellitus showed that an ACE inhibitor (lisinopril) reduced progression of retinopathy in non-hypertensive patients with type 1 diabetes by 50% in 2 years. Currently available evidence supports the use of ACE inhibitors in both hypertensive and non-hypertensive patients with type 1 diabetes to prevent microvascular and macrovascular diabetic complications.

Side effects that limit the use of ACE inhibitors include idiopathic cough and hyperkalaemia, although cough is not observed as often with angiotensin II receptor blockers.

Peripheral autonomic neuropathy is a significant factor contributing to blood pressure lability in diabetic patients. Neurogenic orthostatic hypotension is a common condition in diabetic patients who may suffer varying degrees of light headedness in the mornings after awakening, blurred vision, fatigue, cognitive impairment and headache. In this condition systolic blood pressure falls by 20 mmHg or more and diastolic pressure by 10 mmHg when a patient moves from a supine position to standing. Ways of overcoming this are to drink plenty of fluids, wear support stockings or increase salt intake in the diet. Patients should be advised not to undertake strenuous morning activities, get out of bed or stand up rapidly, avoid excessive heat and avoid drugs which make neurogenic orthostatic hypotension worse, such as beta-blockers and tricyclic anti-depressants.

Nocturnal supine hypertension is less well recognized and more difficult to diagnose. Clinical symptoms are rare but its existence in diabetic patients is of growing concern as evidence now suggests that this condition aggravates nephropathy and may contribute to worsened vision on awakening, which is a common problem in diabetic patients with DR and macular oedema. Factors that contribute to supine hypertension are an increase in circulating blood volume that occurs during the day and the suppression of the renin-angiotensin axis that occurs in the supine position. Ways of trying to reduce its effect are for patients to sleep with their heads raised by 10–15 cm on a pillow, in order to mechanically reduce cranial blood pressure.

Diabetic nephropathy

Diabetic nephropathy is kidney disease that develops in diabetes mellitus and is another microvascular complication of diabetes along with retinopathy. There is a definite association between retinopathy and all levels of abnormal renal function, independent of duration of diabetes and level of glycaemic control, in both types 1 and 2 diabetes, especially in certain ethnic groups.

The commonest way of evaluating renal function is by measuring the urinary albumin excretion rates. In both types 1 and 2 diabetes, renal disease evolves through a stage of normoalbuminuria, progressing to abnormal levels with microalbuminuria and finally to persistent albuminuria (established nephropathy). Traditional measurements of renal function, e.g. urea and creatinine, may well remain normal until well into the established stage of nephropathy (persistent proteinuria). All stages of abnormal renal function with abnormal urinary albumin excretion are associated with increased incidence of DR.

Certainly all patients with refractory retinopathy and macular oedema should have their renal status regularly assessed.

Proteinuria is a known predictor of the development of PDR in type 1 diabetics. In severe proteinuria there is a 95% increased risk of developing diabetic macular oedema among type 1 diabetics. Whether this is due to hyperglycaemia, or if nephropathy truly is an independent risk factor for development of DR, remains uncertain.

Anaemia

Anaemia is a condition which occurs when there is an abnormally low amount of red blood cells which may be due to a number of different causes, including low levels of iron or vitamin B12 in the diet, gastrointestinal bleeding (e.g. duodenal ulcers, tumours) and heavy periods in women. In anaemia haemoglobin levels are typically below 10–11 g/dL. Anaemia often accompanies diabetic kidney disease and is thought to exacerbate the ischaemic aspect of DR. Anaemia in diabetic patients commonly develops during the stage of overt proteinuria but before the onset of even modest renal impairment. Some studies have reported that diabetic patients with haemoglobin levels less than 12 g/dL have a twofold higher prevalence of DR after other known factors have been accounted for and controlled. Severity of retinopathy was directly proportional to the level of anaemia. Among the subjects with retinopathy, the risk of having severe rather than mild DR is five times higher if the haemoglobin levels are less than 12 g/dL. The connection between anaemia and DR is still undergoing further investigation, but the link with progression of nephropathy is now beyond doubt. It is therefore important to aggressively treat anaemia in diabetic patients particularly where there is evidence of nephropathy and/or retinopathy.

Hyperlipidaemia

Evidence suggests that hyperlipidaemia contributes to the progression and morbidity of DR. In the Wisconsin Epidemiologic Study of Diabetic Retinopathy (WESDR), the presence of retinal hard exudates was significantly associated with increased serum cholesterol levels in patients taking insulin. In the Early Treatment Diabetic Retinopathy Study (ETDRS), subjects who had an elevated total cholesterol or low-density lipoprotein cholesterol level were significantly more likely than those with normal levels to have retinal hard exudates. Accumulation of retinal hard exudates can lead to vision loss either from a foveal lipid plaque or from the development of fibrosis. Risks of progressive nephropathy and neuropathy also are reduced with lipid control.

Dyslipidaemia is a recognized risk factor for diabetic renal disease. The WESDR did not report any association between cholesterol levels and the development of diabetic retinopathy and maculopathy. Conversely, the ETDRS demonstrated that raised serum cholesterol and triglycerides are associated with increased hard exudates formation. Raised serum lipid levels also increase the risk of developing subretinal fibrosis which often results in poor vision. Current medical practice is to initiate lipid-lowering therapy on the basis of coronary heart disease risk.

Anecdotally, it has been reported by a number of clinicians that early diabetic maculopathy which presents with just parafoveal streak exudates does improve with the initiation of lipid-lowering statin therapy and there is now evidence to support this. A recent prospective randomized study of 30 diabetic patients with macular oedema and dyslipidaemia found a statistically significant reduction in hard exudates versus controls after initiation of Atorvastatin, although visual acuity was not affected.

Aspirin

The role of aspirin and other anti-inflammatory drugs is an area of current investigation. It has now been shown that diabetic patients have platelets which are more prone to thrombosis. This is thought to be due to increased levels of plasma plasminogen activator inhibitor in diabetics compared with non-diabetics. A recent meta-analysis of all the studies concerning aspirin therapy for other medical indications in the patient with DR neither increases or decreases the risk of development or progression of

DR. Also daily use of aspirin is not associated with increased risk of retinal haemorrhages, vitreous haemorrhage or progression of diabetic macular oedema.

Cigarette smoking

The association between smoking and DR is complex and the effects of smoking on DR seem rather inconsistent. There is however no doubt that smoking is a definite risk factor for other complications of diabetes, in particular cardiovascular disease. Smoking can affect DR in a number of ways by increasing the number of circulating activated leukocytes, causing severe retinal vasoconstriction, increasing lipid levels in smokers and carboxyhaemoglobin-induced hypoxia. Consequently all diabetic patients should be encouraged to not smoke and referred for cessation counselling and advice.

Pregnancy

Pregnancy is a major risk factor for the progression of DR in the short term, but this is typically a transient progression. The long-term risk of progression of DR does not appear to be increased by pregnancy. Altered systemic and retinal haemodynamics seen in pregnancy affect the course of DR with increased retinal blood flow in pregnant women and 6 months thereafter.

The prospective cohort Diabetes in Early Pregnancy Study (DEPS) found that the risk of progression of retinopathy in pregnancy prior to week 14 was increased by elevated HbA1C levels. The increased risk may be caused by a number of factors, namely poor metabolic control or metabolic control which is achieved too rapidly. The recommendation now is that diabetic women should carefully plan their pregnancies as much as possible in order to allow excellent metabolic and blood pressure control to be achieved prior to conception. There are a number of risk factors which affect progression of DR during pregnancy including:

- diabetes duration;
- level of retinopathy at conception;
- blood glucose control;
- co-existing vascular disease and hypertension.

Provided that the diabetic woman in pregnancy is carefully monitored and all systemic disease optimally controlled, the long-term effects on vision can be minimized.

Genetics

Hyperglycaemia and duration of diabetes are important risk factors for the progression of DR. However despite this it is well recognized that some individuals with diabetes who maintain poor control of their diabetes do not develop significant DR even over many years. Conversely other individuals progressively get worsening DR despite maintaining good control of their diabetes. This strongly suggests that there is a genetic factor involved which in some people has a protective effect. Human leukocyte antigen (HLA) studies have found that HLA DR7 may confer resistance to the development of proliferative DR. Currently there are 10 candidate genes that are thought to be associated with DR and many more are likely to be identified in the future. Whether DR has a major genetic basis is still uncertain.

Alcohol

There is no consensus about the effects of alcohol consumption and the development or progression of DR with certain studies producing contradictory evidence.

Obstructive sleep apnoea

Obstructive sleep apnoea (OSA) is a disorder that is relatively common, occurring in approximately 2% of women and 4% of men over the age of 35. It takes its name from the Greek word *apnea*, which means 'without breath'. People with sleep apnoea literally stop breathing repeatedly during their sleep, often for a minute. Sleep apnoea can be caused by either complete obstruction of the airway (obstructive apnoea) or partial obstruction (obstructive hypopnoea involving slow, shallow breathing), both of which can wake one up. There are three types of sleep apnoea: obstructive, central, and mixed. Of these, OSA is the most common.

The exact cause of OSA remains unclear. The site of obstruction in most patients is the soft palate, extending to the region at the base of the tongue. There are no rigid structures, such as cartilage or bone, in this area to hold the airway open. During the day, muscles in the region keep the passage wide open. But as a person with OSA falls asleep, these muscles relax to a point where the airway collapses and becomes obstructed. When the airway closes, breathing stops, and the sleeper awakens to open the airway. The arousal from sleep usually lasts only a few seconds, but brief arousals disrupt continuous sleep and prevent the person from reaching the deep stages of slumber, such as rapid eye movement (REM) sleep, which the body needs in order to rest and replenish its strength. Once normal breathing is restored, the person falls asleep only to repeat the cycle throughout the night.

Typically, the frequency of waking episodes is somewhere between 10 and 60. A person with severe OSA may have more than 100 waking episodes in a single night.

The primary risk factor for OSA is excessive weight gain or obesity. The accumulation of fat on the sides of the upper airway causes it to become narrow and predisposed to closure when the muscles relax. Age is another prominent risk factor. Loss of muscle mass is a common consequence of the aging process. If muscle mass decreases in the airway, it may be replaced with fat, leaving the airway narrow and soft. Men have a greater risk for OSA. Male hormones can also cause structural changes in the upper airway.

OSA is a recognized risk factor for systemic arterial hypertension, pulmonary hypertension as well as nocturnal stroke and myocardial infarction and renal failure, particularly in diabetics.

Anecdotally it has now been suggested that this condition may cause exacerbations of DR with development of more diffuse macular oedema associated with progressive ischaemia. OSA is thought to aggravate DR because of the associated nocturnal recurrent hypoxaemia (inadequate oxygen in the blood) with hypercapnia (where there is excess carbon dioxide in the blood >45 mmHg). The same abnormalities of retinal auto regulation that are induced by hyperglycaemia make the retina susceptible to ischaemic injury from hypoxaemia and hypertension and are made worse by hypercapnia.

In most cases OSA is treated with continuous positive airway pressure (CPAP) or bi-level positive airway pressure (bi-PAP) delivered during sleep by a special nasal mask.

Conclusions

Clinical trials have shown the effectiveness of laser photocoagulation in the prevention of visual loss in moderate to severe DR. It is now becoming increasingly evident that control of other systemic factors and the use of different systemic therapeutic agents are also important in controlling DR progression.

The management of the diabetic patient with DR requires multidisciplinary teamwork between optometrists, general practitioners, ophthalmologists, specialist diabetes nurses, hospital-based physicians and paramedical staff including podiatrists, dieticians and retinal screeners. Only by working together, communicating effectively and also keeping the patient fully informed, will all these systemic factors discussed above be tackled coherently and effectively. The value of good control of diabetes by eating a healthy diet, exercising, smoking cessation and maintaining weight control will all help to reduce the complications caused by diabetes generally.

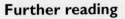

Bergerhoff K, Clar C, Richter B 2002 Aspirin in diabetic retinopathy: a systematic review. *Endocrinology and Metabolism Clinics of North America* **31**: 779–793

Chew E Y, Mills J L, Metzger B E et al 1995 Metabolic control and progression of retinopathy. The diabetes early pregnancy study. National Institute on Child Health and Human Development Diabetes in Early Pregnancy Study. *Diabetes Care* **18**: 631–637

Chowdry T A, Hopkins D, Dodson P M et al 2002 The role of serum lipids in exudative diabetic maculopathy: is there a place for lipid lowering therapy? *Eye* **16**: 689–693

Cusick M, Chew E, Chan C et al 2003 Histopathology and regression of retinal hard exudates in diabetic retinopathy after reduction of elevated serum levels. *Ophthalmology* **110**: 2126–2133

Estacio R O, Jeffers B W, Gifford N et al 2000 Effect of blood pressure control on diabetic microvascular complications in patients with hypertension and type 2 diabetes. *Diabetes Care* **23**: B54–B64

Gupta A, Gupta V, Thapar S et al 2004 The effect of lipid lowering drug Atorvastatin as an adjunct in the management of diabetic macular oedema. *American Journal of Opthalmology* **137**: 675–682

Hogeboom van Buggenum I M, Polak B C P, Reichert-Thoen J W M et al 2002 An angiotensin converting enzyme inhibiting therapy is associated with lower vitreous vascular endothelial growth factor concentrations in patients with proliferative diabetic retinopathy. *Diabetilogia* **45**: 203–209

Klein B E K, Moss S E, Klein R 1990 Effect of pregnancy on progression of diabetic retinopathy. *Diabetes Care* **13**: 34–40

Klein R, Klein B E K, Moss S E et al 1984 The Wisconsin epidemiological study of diabetic retinopathy, III. Prevalence and risk of diabetic retinopathy when age at diagnosis is less than 30 years. *Archives of Ophthalmology* **102**: 520–526, 527–532

Klein R, Klein B E K, Moss S E et al 1988 Glycosylated haemoglobin predicts the incidence and progression of diabetic retinopathy. *Journal of the American Medical Association* **260**: 2864–2871

Klein R, Klein B E K, Moss S E et al 1998 The Wisconsin epidemiologic study of diabetic retinopathy, XVII: the 14 year incidence and progression of diabetic retinopathy and associated risk factors in type 1 diabetes. *Ophthalmology* **105**: 1801–1815

Klein R, Klein B E K 2002 Blood pressure control and diabetic retinopathy. *British Journal Ophthalmology* **86**: 365–367

Loukovaara S, Harju M, Kaaja R et al 2003 Retinal capillary blood flow in diabetic and non diabetic women during pregnancy and post partum period. *Investigative Ophthalmology & Visual Science* **44**: 1486–1491

Mathiesen E R, Ronn B, Storm B et al 1995 The natural course of microalbuminuria in insulin-dependent diabetes: a 10 year prospective study. *Diabetic Medicine* **12**: 482–487

Muhlhauser I, Bender R, Bott U et al 1996 Cigarette smoking and progression of retinopathy and nephropathy in type I diabetics. *Diabetic Medicine* **13**: 536–543

Pradhan R, Fong D, March C et al 2002 Angiotensin-converting enzyme inhibition for the treatment of moderate to severe diabetic retinopathy in normotensive type 2 diabetic patients: A pilot study. *Journal of Diabetes Complications* **16**: 377–381

Radha V, Rema M, Mohan V 2002 Genes and diabetic retinopathy. *Indian Journal of Ophthalmology* **50**: 5–11

Recchia F M, Brown G C 2000 Systemic disorders associated with retinal vascular occlusion. *Current Opinion in Ophthalmology* **11**: 462–467

Retinal Vein Occlusion Guidelines 2004. Online. Available: www.rcophth.ac.uk/docs/publications/RetinalVeinOcclusionGuidelinesMarch2004.pdf

Sen K, Misra A, Kumar A, Pandey R M 2002 Simvastatin retards progression of retinopathy in diabetic patients with hypercholesterolaemia. *Diabetes Research and Clinical Practice* **56**: 1–11

Sinclair S, Delvecchio C, Levin A 2003 Treatment of anemia in the diabetic patient with retinopathy and kidney disease. *American Journal of Ophthalmology* **135**: 740–743

Sinclair S H, Malamut R, Delvecchio C et al 2005 Diabetic retinopathy: Treating systemic conditions aggressively can save sight. *Cleveland Clinic Journal of Medicine* **72**: 447–454

The Diabetes Control and Complications Trial Research Group 1993 The effect of intensive treatment of diabetes on the development and progression of long-term complications in insulin-dependent diabetes mellitus. *New England Journal of Medicine* **329**: 977–986

The Diabetes Control and Complications Trial Research Group 1995 Progression of retinopathy with intensive versus conventional treatment in the diabetes control and complications trial. *Ophthalmology* **102**: 647–661

The Diabetes Control and Complications Trial/Epidemiology of Diabetes and Complications Research Group 2000 Retinopathy and nephropathy in patients with type I diabetes four years after a trial of intensive therapy. *New England Journal of Medicine* **342**: 381–389

The United Kingdom Prospective Diabetes Study Group 1998 Tight blood
pressure control and risk of macrovascular and microvascular complications in
type 2 diabetes. UKPDS Report No 38, *BMJ* **317**: 703–713

The United Kingdom Prospective Diabetes Study Group 1998 Efficacy of atenolol
and captopril in reducing risk of macrovascular and microvascular
complications in type 2 diabetes. *BMJ* **317**: 713–720

Van Leiden H A, Dekker J M, Moll A C et al 2003 Risk factors for incident
retinopathy in a diabetic and nondiabetic population over a 10 year follow up
period. The Hoorn Study. *Archives of Ophthalmology* **121**: 245–251

Index

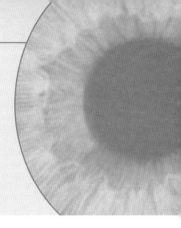